PRAISE FC
EXPLORACISES

"I always look forward to working closely with Betsy Polatin. I greatly appreciate her profound understanding of how our bodies hold trauma and stress in our connective tissues, muscles, and organs, and how to release them through the ingenious exercises, postures, and practices she teaches."

—**Gabor Maté, MD,** author, *The Myth of Normal: Trauma, Illness and Healing in a Toxic Culture*

"*EXPLORACISES®* by Betsy Polatin is a transformative guide that merges body, mind, and spirit. Through her unique approach—Exploracises—Polatin provides exercises that integrate physicality, breathwork, and spiritual practices to foster mental health, creativity, and wellbeing. Focusing on wholeness, tensegrity, fascia, and connection, she invites readers to explore the sacredness of the body and reconnect with the energy of the universe. This book offers powerful tools for healing, self-awareness, and alignment, inspiring a grounded and harmonious life."

—**Stephen Porges, PhD,** author of *The Polyvagal Theory*, creator of the Safe and Sound Protocol (SSP), co-inventor of Sonocea®

"Beautifully written, expansive, and compassionate, EXPLORACISES is an essential resource for restoration and transformation of body, mind, and spirit. This eloquently organized, practical guide reshapes the conversation about the body as a core pathway for healing and transformation. Polatin articulately explains numerous somatic practices that we can immediately apply to gently help us explore and reconnect to ourselves. EXPLORACISES empowers us to reclaim self-agency through movement, rhythm, breath, attunement, enactment, playfulness, curiosity, and synchrony in restoration, recovery, and health."

—**Dr. Cathy Malchiodi**, author of *Trauma and Expressive Arts Therapy: Brain, Body, and Imagination in the Healing Process*

"In this insightful book, Betsy Polatin delves deeper into the marvels of embodiment as it unfolds within relationships, fields of gravity, and the broader universe. She masterfully interweaves the subsystems of tensegrity, the nervous system, and fascia. This brilliant and invaluable resource offers profound support to healing professionals, body-oriented therapists, and anyone seeking to understand their true 'home'—their living, sensing, and knowing body—and its remarkable connection to both heaven and earth."

—**Peter A. Levine, PhD,** author of *An Autobiography of Trauma: A Healing Journey* and *Waking the Tiger: Healing Trauma*

"A bit blown away by the fascia image with the fibres and the water droplets and the similarity to the Energy lines and nodes."

—**Rory Duff**, geobiologist and author, *Grail Found* and *Grail Bound*

"In this brilliant yet practical book, Betsy Polatin guides us in exercises in how to re-member and honor the wisdom of our bodies and the meaning of our synchronized embodiment, reminding us that we are spiritual beings having a human and physical experience. With her wealth of knowledge and experience, she reweaves the unity of Heaven and Earth and our spirituality and embodiment and shows how we can heal and move into wholeness. She then helps us to remember and reconnect with the consciousness and oneness of all of life and guides us in how we can align with that consciousness, wisdom, and love of the Earth and Cosmos and live it in the present moment in an embodied way."

—**Heather Ensworth, PhD,** internationally known astrologer, clinical psychologist, shamanic healer, and co-author of *From Trauma to Healing*

"We live in a time where information comes at a faster rate than we can ever discern, sort, or integrate. Much less tell fact from fiction. The surest way to find our center and bring ourselves into a place of peace is through being present and being in our body. Betsy has pulled together a brilliant 'how to' showing us some very practical, doable and, yes, effective ways to come home to ourselves. This exploration of reconnection to ourselves and our people is simple, gentle, and so welcoming. I am thankful for this invitation to balance the masculine and feminine with myself and thus for us all. I am so excited for us all to find this truth in ourselves and through that journey heal our world at large."

—**Alexsys Thompson,** MLC, BCC, executive coach and best-selling author of *The Power of a Graceful Leader* and *Gratitude Journals*

"'There is more wisdom in your body than in your deepest philosophy.' —**Nietzsche,** *Thus Spoke Zarathustra.* In *EXPLORACISES* we are offered novel insights into the hidden wisdom of the body. In this remarkable book Betsy Polatin brings Nietzsche's famous quote forward to the 21st century with specific advice and exercises teaching us how to access physiological and anatomical systems that lie largely unrecognized in the human body."

—**Sue Carter, PhD,** Distinguished Research Scientist, Executive Director, Emerita, The Kinsey Institute, Indiana University

"*EXPLORACISES*® by Betsy Polatin is a groundbreaking exploration of embodiment, offering a treasure trove of practical exercises that invite deeper connection to body, mind, and breath. Betsy's expert guidance blends science, somatic awareness, and artistry, empowering readers to discover profound calm, resilience, and vitality.

"At Sonocea®, we are passionate about advancing wellbeing through sound, and I see immense synergy between Betsy's work and our mission. Her approach resonates deeply with our understanding of how the nervous system responds to mindful practice, making this book an invaluable resource for anyone seeking transformation and balance in their lives. Whether you're navigating daily stress or supporting others in healing professions, *EXPLORACISES*® will equip you with powerful tools for embodied living.

A must-read for anyone who wants to embody greater presence, ease, and strength."

—**Anthony Gorry,** world-renowned musician and producer, co-inventor of Sonocea®

"Betsy Polatin exhibits a deep well of knowledge and wisdom in the somatics field. Betsy has taken her decades-long passion and has continued to explore, innovate, and integrate not just herself but also the somatics field, as this book clearly shows. I especially found it creative that Betsy does not just have us read about somatics but instead incorporates the body, spirit, and mind with each page one reads. Instead of reading about health and wellbeing, you are somatically experiencing it as you journey through this book."

—**Donnalea Van Vleet Goelz, PhD,** Executive Director of Continuum Movement®, Courtesy Research Assistant Professor at University of Florida College of Medicine, Jacksonville

"Building on the success of her acclaimed book *Humanual*, Betsy once again invites readers to reimagine how we connect with our body, mind, and spirit. This inspiring and comprehensive guide offers profound insights and concepts designed to be seamlessly integrated into everyday life.

"Engaging and practical, the book is infused with wisdom and curiosity, encouraging readers to embrace its meaningful lessons in their daily routines. Through a masterful blend of rich information and experiential exercises, it charts a transformative path toward living in wholeness and embracing the fullness of being human. Whether for personal growth or professional practice, Betsy's latest work serves as a valuable resource for anyone seeking to deepen their understanding of what it means to live in harmony with oneself and the world."

—**Liz Charles, MD,** creator of Sensitive Approach for Safe and Sound Protocol (SSP)

"Betsy shares a deeply felt understanding of her life's work through a unique blend of science, spirituality, and the physical body. She explores a question that many are fascinated with—how we use our body, inhabit it, and move it for health and wellbeing, ultimately connecting with our individual and collective 'why.'

"We must genuinely embody knowledge to reach simplicity. Betsy grounds the complex and abstract topics of spirituality, healing, emotions, and trauma in the physicality of our body—our movements, rhythms, breath, fascia, and vagus nerve. She guides us into our own physicality through helpful metaphors, intentional acts, conscious movements, and pragmatic exercises. It's profoundly evident that Betsy holds everything she teaches us within her own body, breath, movement, presence, and daily practice.

"We often attach spirituality to an out-of-body or larger-than-life experience. We utilize spirituality as a resource for coping with the uncertainty, chaos, and challenge of living on this earthly planet. In a way, this type of spirituality takes us out of our bodies and disconnects us from one another.

"In contrast, Betsy grounds spirituality in our physicality—our breath, our movements, our fascia. Betsy's approach combining science, spirituality, and on-the-ground practices is rooted in our physiology. She provides us with not only a way to manage the inherent pains and struggles of modern life, but a pragmatic pathway of deepening connection with ourselves, one another, and the world we live in."

—**Michael Allison**, Polyvagal Performance Consultant, Educational Partner, Polyvagal Institute, and founder of The Play Zone

EXPLORACISES®

Heaven and Earth Meet in Synchronized Embodiment

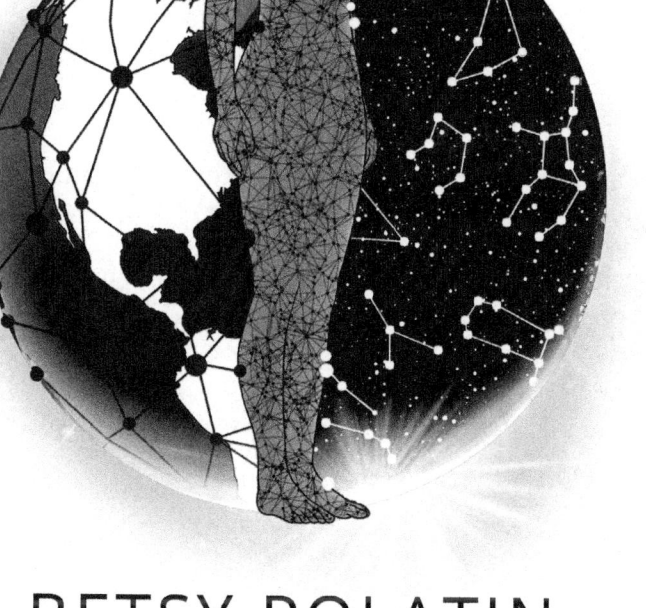

BETSY POLATIN

Copyright © 2025 by Betsy Polatin.
All rights reserved. This book or any portion thereof may not be reproduced or used in any manner whatsoever without the express written permission of the publisher except for the use of brief quotations in a book review.

Publishing Services provided by Paper Raven Books LLC
Printed in the United States of America
First Printing, 2025

ISBN 979-8-9928340-0-0

EXPLORACISES is dedicated to:

The depth of human heart and soul that universally connects us all, amidst the shattering.... heralding the Age of Aquarius. Uni-Verse as One-Song.

ACKNOWLEDGMENTS

Thank you to Stephen Porges, PhD, for his continued support of my work, and for his generosity in answering my questions. Thank you to Dr. Aline LaPierre for her depth of understanding, and her wonderful NeuroAffective Touch work. Thank you to Heather Ensworth, PhD, for her insights, videos, and information, and to Rory Duff for his ley line drawings and his wonderful teachings.

—Much gratitude to Peter Levine, PhD, for the joy of teaching "Trauma and The Performing Artist" together, and for being my teacher, mentor, and colleague for 25 years. Thank you, Dr. Gabor Maté, for the pleasure and adventure of co-teaching with you these past few years. Always grateful to Richard Schwartz, PhD, and Dr. Bessel van der Kolk, longtime champions of trauma healing work. Thank you for the informative videos: Gil Hedley, PhD; Tom Myers; Robert Holden, PhD; Caroline Myss; Pam Gregory; BiotensegriTea Party. Thank you all for sparking my imagination and igniting my creativity.

—Thank you to Kathy Glass for the brilliant editing and advice. Huge thank-you to Chris Ouellette for all the beautiful and breathtaking illustrations, and to Krystal Chryssomallis for the lovely back cover photograph. Thanks to Morgan, Megan, Julia, and the wonderful team at Paper Raven books. Extra-special thanks and hugs to Daria and Ruby, my amazing daughters, and Axel, Vaughn, and Logan, my wonderful grandsons. Thank you to the unseen world, that wraps me in golden white light and gives me the courage to go on.

FOREWORD

EXploracises

This book is about saying YES to the physicality of life.

In a world where it is tempting to turn away from our bodies, where enhancing ourselves with silicon-based consciousness seems appealing to some, Betsy invites us to inquire deeply into the organic experience of bodily sensations as they work in collaborative unity with mindful awareness and spiritual presence.

Following Betsy's precise inquiry process, I felt a growing excitement stir. A choir of voices arose: *Someone knows we exist! Someone is talking to ME!* My bio-intelligent story was being called out of the shadows. Finally, my body was honored as essential, and my DNA was directly spoken to.

Betsy guides us into a world where the movement of the body is one and the same as the mind's thought. Her YES to life is broad and deep. She helps us discover our stunning biological design and stimulates a felt-sense excitement at the recognition of the complex, multidimensional beings we are today. She prepares us for inevitable becoming.

Walking the EXploracise path, I experienced that coming home to my body is remembering the extraordinary evolutionary journey we all took to master living on this planet. I realized that beyond my personal childhood, my body had a childhood too—one that is anchored to life as it began on this planet. A homecoming that brought awe and gratitude.

But homecoming demands participation, a turning towards which each EXploracise expertly invites. EXploracises aim to reduce limiting beliefs. They prompt us to ask different questions of ourselves and demand that body, mind, and spirit enter into a collaborative relationship few of us think to establish.

Our human ability to override, mask, appease, or hide in functional freeze, all the while giving the appearance of normalcy, is well-honed. Although Betsy offers EXploracises that may help with grounding, self-regulation, or coping strategies, her work is not about simply adding more tools to the toolbox. It is about demystifying the laws of biological intelligence.

All very well. But it's natural to contract in the face of difficulty, and difficulty is not in short supply. Isn't the body a source of pain? Of discontent? Of constant tending? Why should I go there? And what does it mean to say YES to life these days?

Betsy suggests a new paradigm of physicality in which *synchronized embodiment* gives us the opportunity to see the total pattern of our experience and do something lasting about it. A paradigm shift where our relationship to ourselves includes developing *kinesthetic intelligence* and coherent *fascial biotensegrity* to maintain dynamic balance. This may sound esoteric, but the point of EXploracises is to walk us through experiences that lift the mystery and empower us

FOREWORD

to shape our own bodies—not only our physical body, but since they function as one, our mental, emotional, and spiritual bodies as well.

Betsy works on the premise that our physicality develops based on how we do things. Our bodies grow based on how we use them, therefore, creating the right conditions is key. She clearly walks us through the vast and varied therapeutic implications of moving with inner organization. In other words, it's never too late to learn new ways, and it has been her life's work to lay down a path we can follow to reliably do so.

Dr. Aline LaPierre

Founder, *The NeuroAffective Touch Institute,*
Coauthor, *Healing Developmental Trauma,*
President, *The United States Association for Body Psychotherapy,*
Editor-in-Chief, *The International Body Psychotherapy Journal*

PREFACE

HUMANUAL presents *EXPLORACISES*

Welcome to a presentation of the body as something integrated rather than separate from personhood. Welcome to the inspiration that brings a very different sense of how we can enter into deeper relationship with ourselves. Welcome to the uplifting concept of tensegrity, uniting us with the greater cosmos. Welcome to the wonder and immediacy of Heaven and Earth meeting in synchronized embodiment.

This book expands on the simple but profound concepts and exploratory movements introduced in *HUMANUAL*, with a more free-flowing form of exploration that I call "EXploracises." The presentation and the practices are lighter and often open-ended. I hope they are also inviting and accessible. For those who want more concrete detail, information, and explanations, please read *HUMANUAL, An Epic Journey to your Expanded Self*. It poses and suggests some answers to the following questions: "Each of us has an everyday self that we assume our self to be. But what if there is more to us than meets the

EXPLORACISES

eye? What if there is an *expanded* version of our self that includes not only the habitual patterns, the lost parts, and the innate organization but also a connection to the grand, scintillating space of the universe and the possibilities it offers us?" On to *EXploracises*.

To use this book you can either read it in the order it was written, as it does follow a logical (to me) sequence, or you can read and do the EXploracises in any order. Pick the book up any time and select what is of interest or relevance to you, perhaps to match what is happening in your life.

Sometimes it may seem like "EXs" are randomly suggested, but in truth they are inextricably connected. There is an EX for the tongue followed by an EX for the shoulder. It is not random because there is a muscle called the omohyoid that goes from the shoulder to the hyoid bone, near the base of the tongue. And if we stay consistent with the unity and oneness point of view, our concepts merge with the image and reality of the fascial system, where everything is in fact materially and energetically connected to everything else.

After every EX when something has changed, you always want to integrate that change or sensation into the rhythm of the whole system. Otherwise it may not last or remain accessible. The new energy must be welcomed at all levels. If we consider our whole physicality to be 100 percent, then an injury in the arm might be 5 percent. Even if you "fix" the injury, the other 95 percent is still in the pattern of what caused the injury. So, integrating your innate rhythm and wholeness invites more flow and life force to your system. The EXploracises will help you do this.

Off you go with a sense of wonder at the synchronicities, complexities, and magnificence of life. An appreciation for contact, a smile, or just communication. A recognition of the injustice, and the suffering. And remember the children, such blessed beings, here at this unique time of transformation on the planet. Youthful, innocent faces,

PREFACE

all over the world, all looking up at the same sky. It is said that the longest journey is the one from your head to your heart. Let's embark on that journey together.

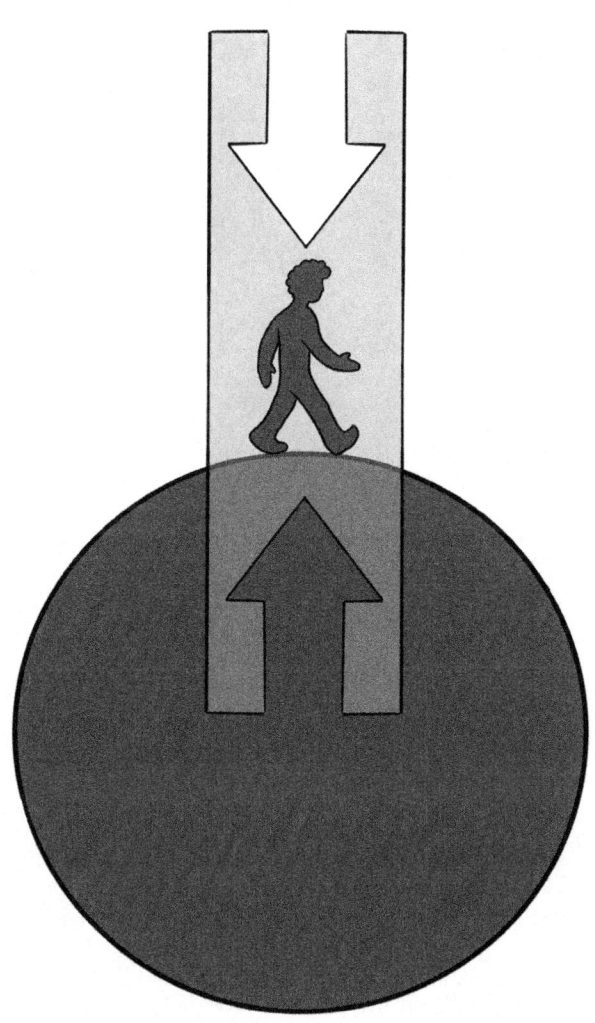

CONTENTS

INTRODUCTION 1

Chapter 1 – WHOLENESS, TENSEGRITY, AND FASCIA 7

I – WHOLENESS AND UNITY 8

II – TENSEGRITY. 11

III – BIOTENSEGRITY 15

IV – FASCIA 18

V – FASCIA AND MOVEMENT 25

VI – PANDICULATION 31

Chapter 2 – HEAVEN AND EARTH MEET in SYNCHRONIZED EMBODIMENT 35

I – UNIVERSAL LAWS OF PHYSICALITY. 36

II – COHERENCE. 41

III – UNIVERSAL FORCES FROM HEAVEN AND EARTH. 45

IV – SPIRALS 52

V – Being in the PRESENT MOMENT or Having PRESENCE 61

Chapter 3 – PHYSICALITY 65
I – INTRODUCTION TO PHYSICALITY. 66
II – SPECIFICS OF PHYSICALITY 73
III – BODY MAP 77
IV – SOMATIC PRINCIPLES 86
V – NUANCES OF PHYSICALITY 94
VI – SUSPENSION 104
VII – SUPPORT 107

Chapter 4 – TAKING EXPLORACISES TO THE NEXT LEVEL. 117
I – DEEPER DIVE EXPLORACISES 118
II – SIMPLE MOVEMENT EXPLORACISES. 120
III – MULTILEVEL EXPLORACISES. 125

Chapter 5 – BREATH. 147
I – INTRODUCTION TO BREATH 148
II – BREATHING EXPLORACISES 152

Chapter 6 – HEART 175
I – INTRODUCTION TO THE HEART 176
II – HEART EXPLORACISES 181

Chapter 7 – SPIRIT and MEDITATION 189
I – INTRODUCTION TO SPIRITUALITY 190
II – MEDITATION EXPLORACISES 195

Chapter 8 – EMOTION. 207
I – INTRODUCTION TO EMOTION 208
II – EMOTION EXPLORACISES. 210

III – ANGER 218
IV – ANXIETY 220
V – FEAR 224
VI – LOVE 226

Chapter 9 – THE VAGUS NERVE AND THE POLYVAGAL THEORY 231
I – INTRODUCTION TO THE VAGUS NERVE 232
II – POLYVAGAL EXPLORACISES 235
III – HUMANUAL POLYVAGAL SMILE 239

Chapter 10 – TRAUMA 243
I – INTRODUCTION TO TRAUMA 244
II – TRAUMA EXPLORACISES 247
III – ANATOMICAL FACTS RELATED TO TRAUMATIC RESPONSES 252

Chapter 11 – PERFORMANCE 267
I – INTRODUCTION TO PERFORMANCE 268
II – ACTING 271
III – MUSIC 277
IV – TAKING THE STAGE 287

Chapter 12 – WE IS THE NEW ME 291

ENDNOTES 315
ABOUT THE AUTHOR 323

Note – No part of this book was written with AI.

INTRODUCTION

This book is a tribute to the physicality that we all have in this lifetime. Whether we evolved from animals, or we came from the galactic universe, or we emerged from the ocean, if you are reading this, you have a body, and you are here. Bodily sensations meet mindful awareness and spiritual presence. We are an amazing and profound mixture of times gone by and times to come and of course the powerful present moment.

Looking at our past, we see that our ancestors' DNA, energetic patterns, and traits live strong in our desires and choices. Looking toward our future, we realize that our present-day behavior decides our habits, and our habits decide our future. Looking at the present moment, the moment we belong to, we see hopes and dreams, smiles and schemes, rocks and streams, comings and goings. As we look at spiritual realms, we can intuit that we are divine beings having an earthly experience. Our heavenly soul self is having an earthly human experience—Heaven and Earth meeting in synchronized embodiment.

EXPLORACISES

I want to bring Heaven to Earth and Earth to Heaven. The way we do that is through our human body, mind, and spirit. Human uprightness connects us to the Earth below and the Heavens above. Some people think of Heaven as feminine, light, airy, floating free. And the Earth as masculine, solid, contact, dark, and strong. Others see it the other way around: the Heavens, the sun, as the masculine, strong, ruling, and powerful, and the Earth as the feminine, receptive, nurturing, and available. I don't think it matters what your point of view is. Both Heaven and Earth are there in all of us one way or another, and our physicality is our way of connecting, recognizing, and respecting both.

There is room for freedom, nonlinear directions, imagination, metaphor, symbols, and the unseen. And there is also room for matter, manifestation, solidity, stability, and the practical. Both. What would life be without the whimsical, the silk scarf in the wind, the dreams, the free flow, the wonder, and the seeker? Yet we also seem to need the linear, the logical, the rules, directions, limits, deadlines, commitments, and order. The sacred masculine and the sacred feminine in an entwined balance of frequency, vibration, and energy. We embrace and explore it all. The practices, somatic meditations, and contemplations presented in these pages are about exploration, so they are called "EXPLORACISES" or EX for short.

INTRODUCTION

EX – Heart Breath

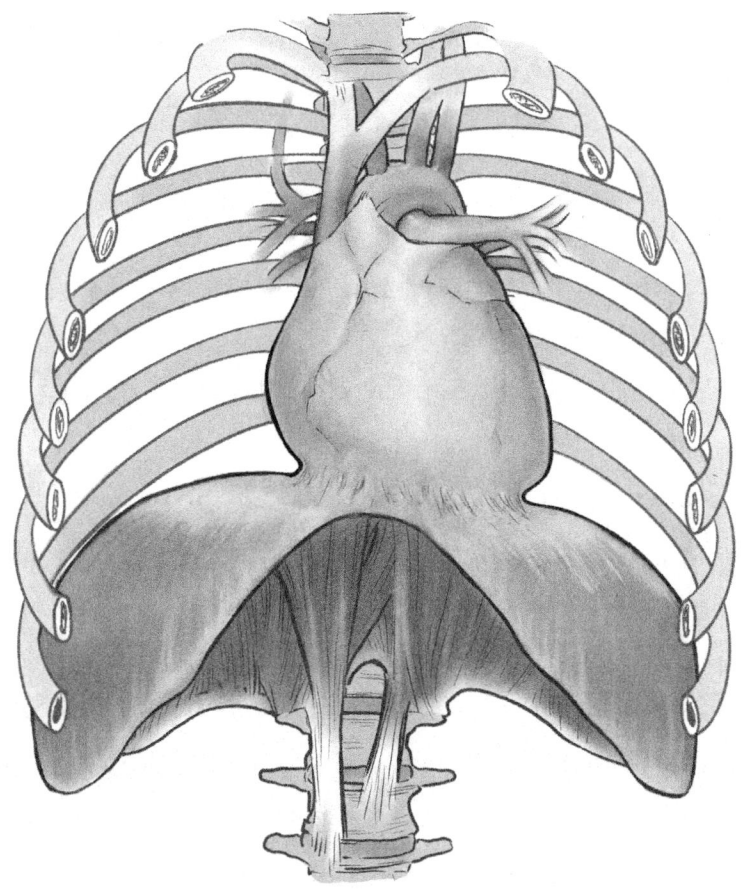

Heart and Diaphragm

1. Breath connects to heart. Your breath connects to your heart.
2. Air flows into your physical being, and your dome-shaped diaphragm glides up and down in rhythm, your rhythm, your rhythm of this moment.
3. This movement ripples through your being, creating shape changes, thought changes, spiritual and perceptual changes.

EXPLORACISES

4. Your heart is tucked in, to the side of your left lung, and it also sits on your diaphragm, the dome-shaped muscle/organ of respiration.
5. Notice that every breath you take touches, moves, and vibrates your heart.
6. Your heart holds freedom, ecstasy, and joy and/or pain, shame, and sorrow. They sit side by side and share the space of your heart. And your breath flows through all of it.
7. Your breath moves your heart.
8. As the air flows through, the concrete walls that you built can crumple, and the protection can be questioned.
9. Like opening a window on the first spring day after a long winter.
10. The pain and the joy or the Heaven and Earth or masculine and feminine intertwine, like vines growing together.
11. Put one hand on your chest and feel the movement of your breath, your rhythm, your hard-earned rhythm.
12. Every note of your song is a glimpse of your life, harmonizing in this moment. The song of the spheres.
13. Feel your hand rise and fall.
14. Honor your journey, whatever it may be.

INTRODUCTION

EX – Choose Your Path

1. Instead of living in fear and trying to figure everything out—politics, COVID, climate change, inflation, war:
2. Hold doors for others.
3. Let people cut in front of you in traffic.
4. Keep babies entertained in grocery lines.
5. Stop and talk to someone who is lonely.
6. Tip generously.
7. Share food.
8. Give children a thumbs-up.
9. Be patient with sales clerks who don't speak your language.
10. Smile at a passerby.
11. Cultivate understanding, and judge less.
12. Be kind to a stranger.
13. Give grace to people who may be having a bad day.
14. Be forgiving with yourself.
15. This is Heaven and Earth meeting in synchronized embodiment.

We is the new me. We are deeply connected to ourselves, and to each other. It is not just our cell phones that have connection, to our cars and computers… but we have a biological longing to connect to each other. This is especially true for children. Our Earth flies around the cosmos, while the clouds embrace the wind in the soft blue sky. The breeze blows the magnificent molecules of manna, given so freely in each moment. Watch, embrace, allow the breeze to set your breath free. Wind chimes tinkling in the softly moving air, the silk scarf blown by the wind, water through sand, porous. Every opening, receiving and giving back. Softer than soft and stronger than strong, never ending, for now. Amidst the gunshots, blasts, tears and fears, a holy, sacred unity struggles to survive. Its fabric is torn, frayed, and dirty from human neglect. But it will never give up. Some humans will die, others will live, and Heaven and Earth will go on. I hope we can be there.

> "Earth's crammed with heaven,
> And every common bush afire with God,
> But only he who sees takes off his shoes;
> The rest sit round and pluck blackberries."
>
> *—Elizabeth Barrett Browning*

CHAPTER 1

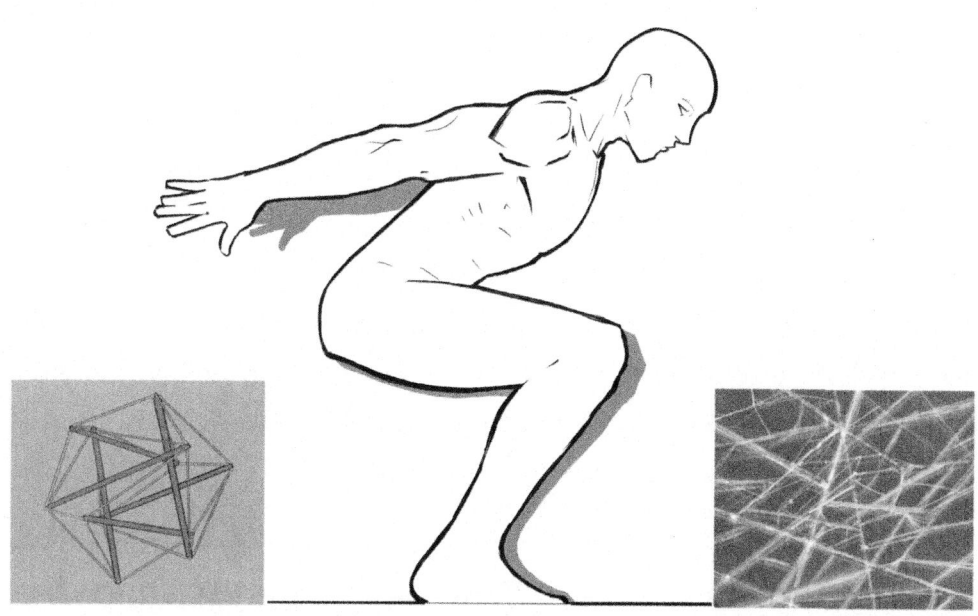

WHOLENESS, TENSEGRITY, AND FASCIA

I – WHOLENESS AND UNITY

Let's start with the beginning we all had: a single cell. The cell, of course, went on to divide, and grow, and split, and twist, and form pathways, tubes, and tunnels, and soft bits, and then hard bits to protect the soft bits, and more. It looks like a bunch of separate components, but it is essentially one entity. No physical parts, just distinctions. It is something like this next EXploracise.

EX – Vendor in the Park Who Sells Animal Balloons

1. He blows up one big balloon.
2. He twists it and forms a head.
3. Twists it again and makes legs, and again for a tail.
4. It ends up looking like a dog.
5. The parts look very different from the whole balloon.

I – WHOLENESS AND UNITY

6. Same with us. Our wholeness or unity is there, no matter how many different aspects we see. Arms and legs are not separate appendages—just one whole balloon self.
7. These generative forces of growth and development of an embryo are the same as the regenerative forces that help you heal back to health and wholeness later in life.
8. Paying attention to how you move can positively direct this process.

EX – Movement Wholeness

1. People talk about wholeness, but do you actually believe it enough to move as a whole unit?
2. When you pick up a book, do you realize that all of you is involved in the activity, and the whole of you changes shape?
3. If not, you will be straining, and one part of you will do the majority of the work. Having one part doing the work is not efficient or holistic.

EX – Antagonistic Pairs

1. Separately strengthening individual muscles and thinking of muscles only working in antagonistic pairs is an outdated model of movement.
2. The common belief: Hamstrings and quadriceps are said to be antagonistic pairs, meaning that as one works, the other will let go.

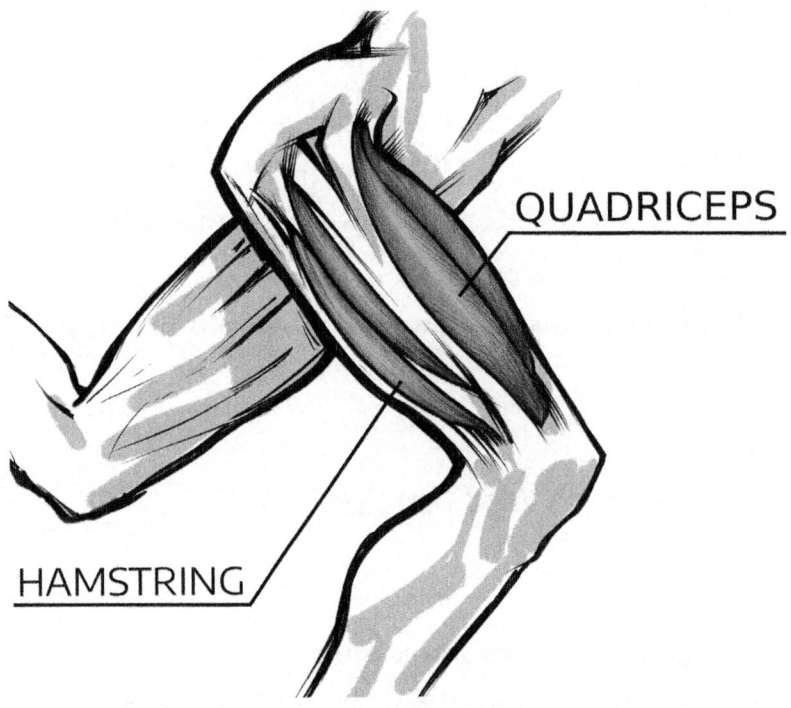

Hamstring and Quadriceps

3. Sit and put one hand on the front of your leg and one hand on the back.
4. Stand and feel which muscles work.
5. They both do! It is not only one muscle working and one letting go. All muscles are involved, some more, some less.

Presently, the less-informed picture of human functional movement is that we are like bricks stacked up and have hanging limbs on a skeleton moved by lever muscles in antagonistic pairs. Nothing could be farther from the truth. Because in that model, we are ignoring the form and function of the layer of connective tissue that surrounds all the muscles as a unified web or net. This brings us to the tensegrity model.[1]

II – TENSEGRITY

The word *tensegrity* is a combination of the words *tension* and *integrity*. The concept was invented by Kenneth Snelson, an innovative artist and sculptor, and later the word was popularized by Buckminster Fuller, the architect who designed the geodesic dome. Tensegrity is a balance of forces that reach a stable but dynamic equilibrium. It manifests when a continuous web of forces is pulling in, counterbalanced by noncontinuous forces pushing out. In our human tensegrity-like model, the large web of connective tissue pushes in while the bones push out. Our bodies are organized by this one continuous connective tissue called a *fascial web*, a living, liquid-gel, shimmering, elastic web. This web forms a tensile structure while the bones that are suspended and balanced within the web of tension push out against it. You do not actually see a tensegrity structure in the human form, but you can feel the dynamic pushes and pulls. The map is not the territory.

EXPLORACISES

The illustration below is a tensegrity icosahedron model. It's called an icosahedron because if you add strings between the ends of every parallel strut, you get 20 nearly equal triangles (the icosahedron) as its faces, 30 edges, and 12 vertices.

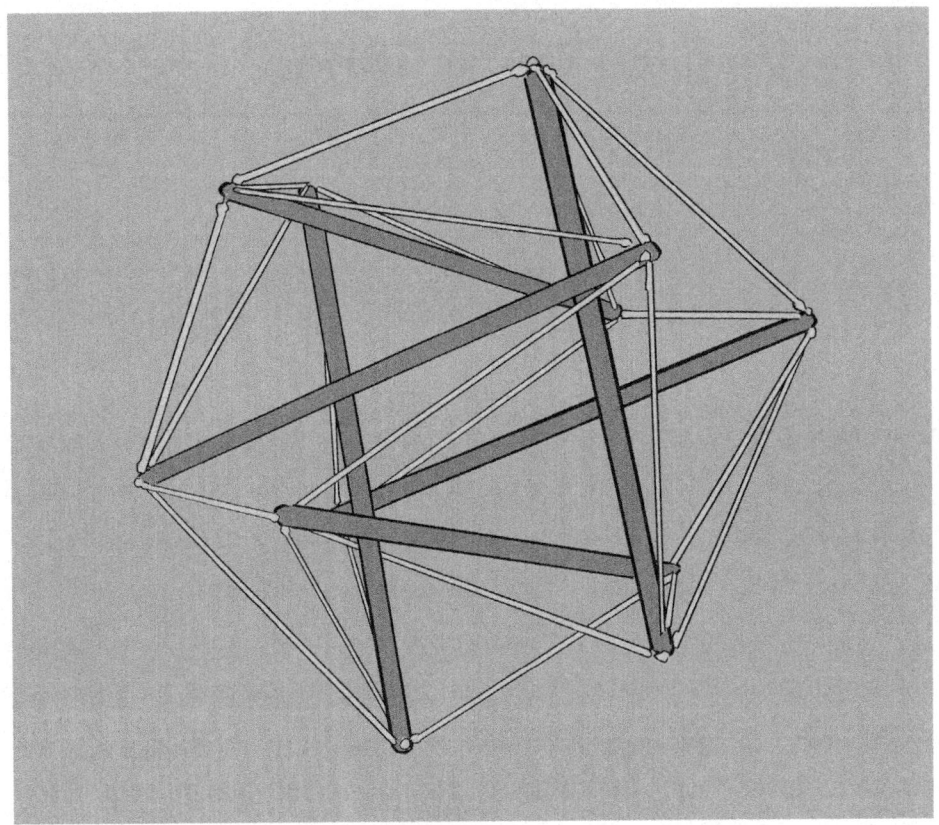

Tensegrity Model

EX – Tensegrity Wholeness

1. Picture this: Since tensegrity is a continuous tensional network, changes in one part are evenly and widely distributed through the whole network. Impact in one part will immediately be distributed globally.

II - TENSEGRITY

2. For example, when you bump your arm, it is not just your arm that feels it—your whole body absorbs the blow. Whatever happens in one part is adapted to by the whole body, a global system from head to toe.

3. If you add a large weight by picking up a heavy object, like a plant or your child, the weight is distributed globally and managed by the whole system, making it much easier to handle. Because weight is being distributed, it prevents force from accumulating at one spot, which could manifest as a problem.

4. If one part of you is out of balance, everything is out of balance, like if you stand with most of your weight on one foot. If imbalance is maintained for an extended period of time, it can cause discomfort or injury.

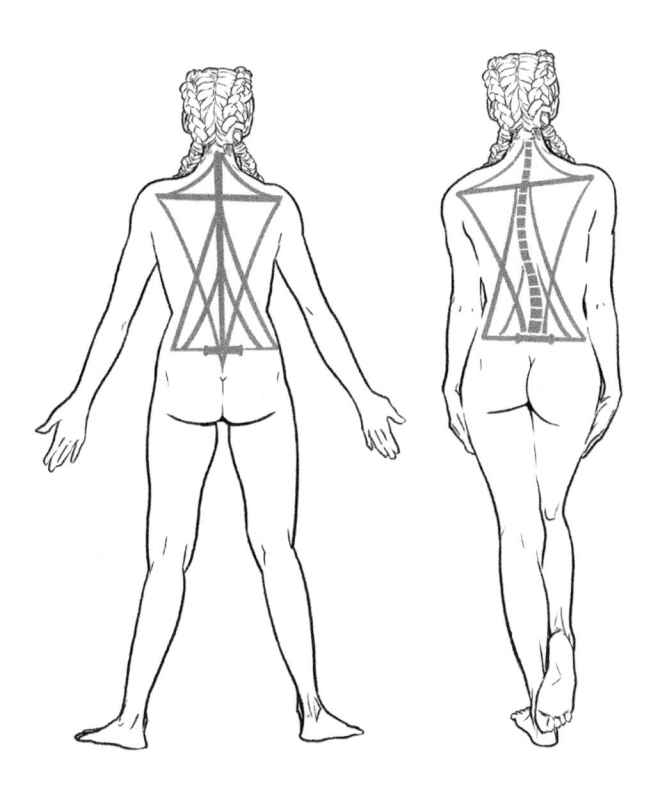

Standing in and out of balance

EX – Tensegrity Fingertip Movement

1. Stand in a comfortable position with your arms by your sides.
2. Let your hands rest with open palms and free wrists, as part of the global tensional network. Your hands will be slightly cupped.
3. Begin to move your fingertips into the space around you.
4. Add your hand and arm.
5. Notice that as soon as you move your arm, your ribs also move, and your hips and legs slightly adjust. Also notice that if you are tightening anywhere, there will be less movement.
6. Allow your whole body to move. Don't brace one part to get another part to move.
7. Continue moving your fingertips into the space around you. Pierce the space with your fingertips. You may notice that this movement invites a breath.

III – BIOTENSEGRITY

The term *biotensegrity* (bio = all living) was coined by Dr. Stephen Levin, an orthopedic surgeon. Dr. Levin could not make sense of the lever/muscle, mechanistic model applied to humans—or animals, for that matter. Look at an image of the classic dinosaur (the sauropod). With the lever model the long-necked creature would topple over.

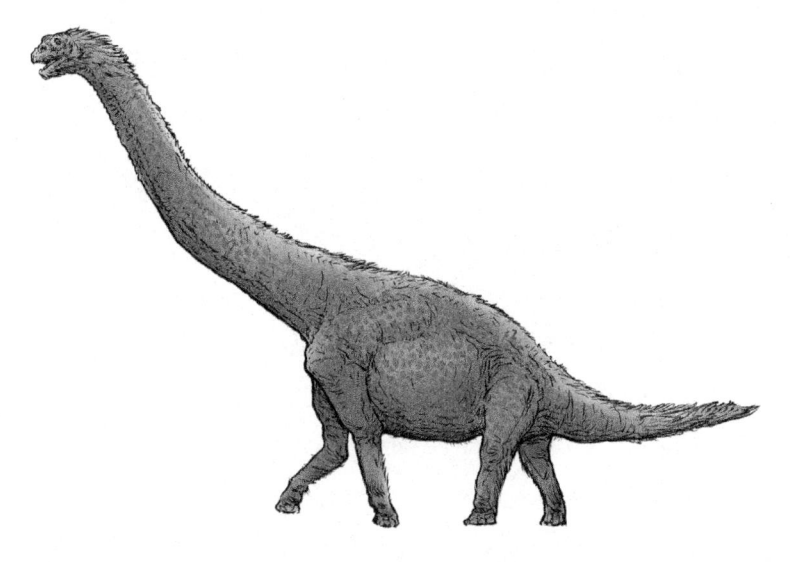

Sauropod Dinosaur

But the tensegrity model explained how that neck could be part of a whole integrated system of the fascial web and the bones, as explained above. The field of biotensegrity is a natural evolution from the study of tensegrity. It explores how tensegrity manifests in biological systems—from viruses and cells, to tissues, to whole living systems. It is a model or a map; it is not exactly the actual thing. The biotensegrity model for human biology is millions of years old, in contrast to the mechanistic machine model applied to humans, which is relatively new.

EX – Biotensegrity Principles (that are helpful to us as living and moving creatures)

1. One part moves, everything moves.
2. Constriction in one place prevents flow in all.
3. Every part is essential and needed.
4. Each part is as important as the next.
5. Lightness and weightlessness are possible to feel.
6. The physical body has an innate springy/elastic quality.
7. Bones do not touch each other directly.

EX – Sesamoid Bones

1. Sesamoid bones are bones that float, meaning they are not attached to anything.
2. Dr. Levin said, "All bones are sesamoid bones."[2]
3. Can you picture all your bones floating?

III – BIOTENSEGRITY

4. It will be helpful to remember that the fascial web of connective tissue keeps the floating in a manageable range, bones and soft tissue working together, in unity.

The biotensegrity model includes healing strategies that resolve individual structural problems and guide the system back toward resilience and greater potential. When we remove restrictions in one part, the whole system has the potential to open. For example, a tight hip will restrict your arm movement for your tennis swing. Releasing the muscles and fascia in your hip will allow your arm to swing freely. Could biotensegrity principles become the new biomechanics? Healing takes place naturally when we remove what is in the way of the healing (often tight muscles and fascia). The body heals itself…if the conditions are right.

IV – FASCIA

Fascia is not a newly discovered tissue, but it has been ignored by anatomists for many years. They were interested in muscles and so they cut the fascia away, thinking it did not matter. But now they are discovering the amazing properties of fascia and the functions it serves.

In the human body, we have a fascial system made up of collagen and elastin fibers. Fascia is a thin casing of connective tissue that surrounds and holds every organ, blood vessel, bone, nerve fiber, and muscle in place. The fascial web is an intricate, continuous, three-dimensional web with tubes and tunnels, the matrix of structural support. This multidirectional, multidimensional fascial arrangement allows you to move in multiple directions. Fascia is one type of connective tissue in a family that has many members. All fascia is connective tissue, but NOT all connective tissue is fascia.

Cells begin creating fascia starting on day 15 after conception, and the tissues continue to grow and multiply. If you look at a body without skin, you see muscle and fascia everywhere. The fascia comprises an

IV – FASCIA

elastic suit or envelope covering almost everything, including bones, muscles, cartilage, and organs. Every bit of you is connected to other bits of you. No parts, only distinctions. One unified connected entity that is interdependent and independent. The unitary system is present in us from top to bottom, and from birth to death.

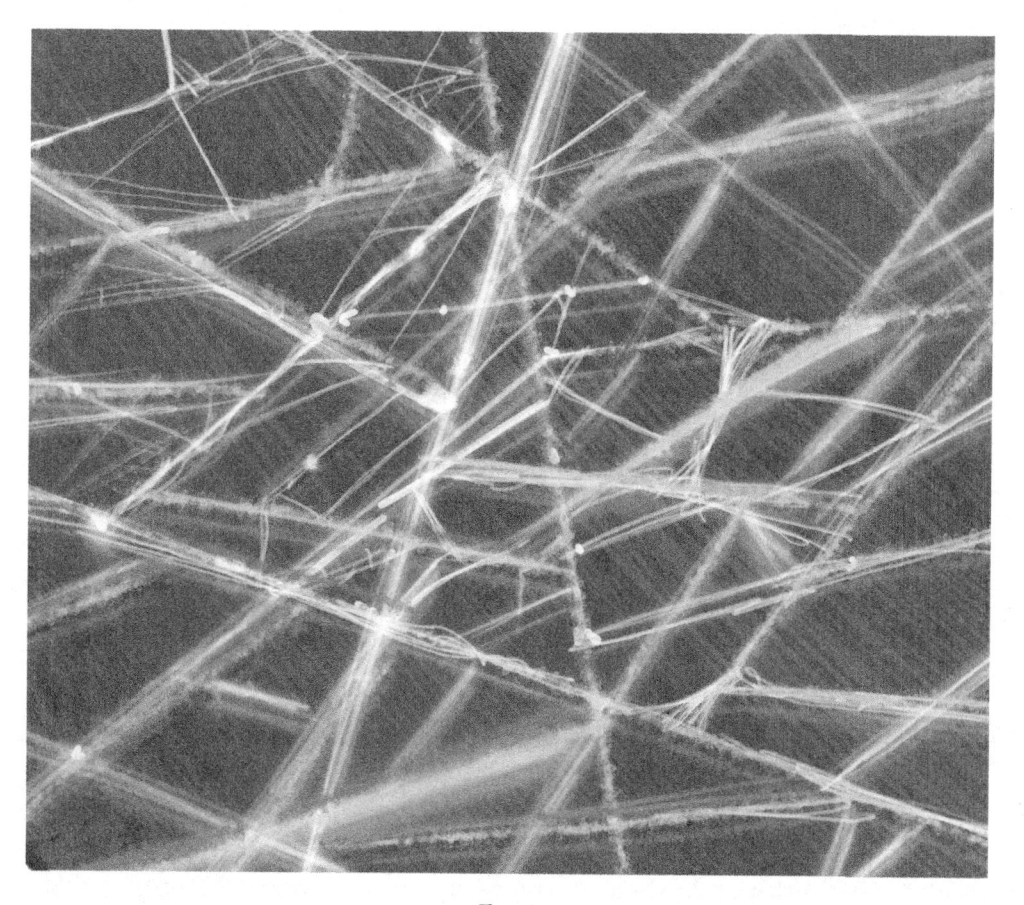

Fascia

EXPLORACISES

EX – Elastic Suit

1. Start sitting in a chair, feet on the ground.
2. Become aware that just under the skin of your whole body is a thin layer of fascia. It is like you are wearing an elastic suit. Twist to one side, then let go, and you will see that you bounce back to center. Or, even simpler, bend one finger back, let go, and watch it spring back.
3. Notice if there are some parts where the elastics have become overstretched and flaccid, and some parts where they have become rigid or even brittle.
4. Then slowly begin to pivot forward and back from your hip joints. Move slowly enough to be aware that the elastic suit has to change shape as you move.
5. You may notice your foot contact changing, the muscles in your back may change, or your breath may change, as your elastic suit adapts to your changing landscape.

The fascial fibers of your elastic suit contain about 70 percent water. The body as a whole is made up of almost 90 percent water, molecularly. Did you ever wonder why the water doesn't just drop down to your legs and feet to look like water balloons? The answer is the fascial net or web that wraps every part of you in every other part of you. The biological fabric of the body can be likened to an orange with its sections. You can see the larger container of orange skin with a white fibrous inner coat, then smaller pieces in a section, and liquid drops in a small membrane. Oranges, and we, are composed of tightly packed bags of water, all communicating with each other, creating a webwork of soft tissue, connecting everything. We see a biceps muscle and think it exists on its own. But in truth, it has relationships up and down and side to side with neighboring tissue. In the USA, we have ZIP codes, but it is still one large country, not really separated by the codes.

The fascia is the largest sensory organ, like a giant satellite dish. It connects all systems, including skeletal, muscular, and more. The tissue does more than provide internal structure; fascia has nerves that make it almost as sensitive as skin. There are six times more nerve endings in fascia than in muscle, and it has 250 million sensory neurons, providing information to proprioception, or the sense of what is happening in one's own body. From this view we can ask: Do we have 600 separate muscles or one large muscle separated by 600 fascial clusters?

EX – Simple Ways to Release Fascia

1. Touch your tongue to the inside of your cheeks. Release.
2. Put your hand about half an inch in front of your mouth and blow on your exhale. Stop.
3. Stick your tongue out as far as you can to release the back of your throat.
4. Equate the fascial elasticity with a musical string on a guitar or violin. When it has the right amount of tautness, the string vibrates in a harmonious way, with a pleasant frequency. If the elastics or strings are too taut or too loose, the sound is off. Same with our fascia. Imagine your fascia as musically tuned strings. The strings of musical instruments used to be made from animal innards.

EXPLORACISES

You can feel the first layer of the fascial system by picking up the skin on your arm. Under that is a thicker, more shaped layer, and under that is the "plastic wrap" layer, around muscles and bones. (For those of you who prepare chicken, fascia is the white elastic layer you see.) We tend to distinguish the layers, but it is a unitary system, a gel-like fluid that slides and glides. For many reasons, including stress, the system can get dried out or overused, or inflamed, and then it sticks together and does not slide or glide, and injury and/or discomfort are sure to follow. Fascia builds more slowly than muscles, so if you are injured, be sure to give the fascia time to heal.

EX – Nervous System and Fascial System

1. You can choose to respond with your fascial system, not your nervous system. The nervous system will give information, but you choose how you respond.
2. When you have an anxious thought about something you have to do, and your stomach tenses…
3. In a split second, evaluate the event and access the nerve endings in the fascial system. Bring your attention to your whole elastic suit, and see if that doesn't relieve some of the anxiety. Picture the illustration of the fascia coursing through your whole body.

IV – FASCIA

EX – Our Fascial Self

1. Fascia is the fabric of our soul. Let yourself discover this living liquid-crystalline web of your bio-intelligence. If we imagine a crystal in liquid form, this would be a metaphorical description of the shimmering fascia.
2. Begin to move slowly and mindfully to know yourself as this body.
3. Let the flow begin to move you.
4. This is the aspect of yourself that loves to move and flow through the air, perhaps singing and dancing, or at least humming, awakening, and enlivening.
5. Feel your energy moving through the network of you. We sense this as the energetic body, vibrating in your frequency.
6. Sense if any energy gets stuck or collapses as you move in this flowing way.
7. If you have the opportunity, do this when you are out in nature, and elicit the help of the trees or ocean.

Some say fascia is your soul, the living web of liquid-crystalline matrix, a superconductor that drives, weaves, and adapts the tensional and compression forces of our bodies and our lives. This happened, and you grew this way, your bio-intelligent story. The fascial system shows it all. And if we extend it out, fascia co-regulates us with each other, with nature, and with a grand web of consciousness and light. The fascial system will connect the world. The body keeps the score, but it is said that fascia is the referee. It calls the shots with 250 million sensory neurons.

EXPLORACISES

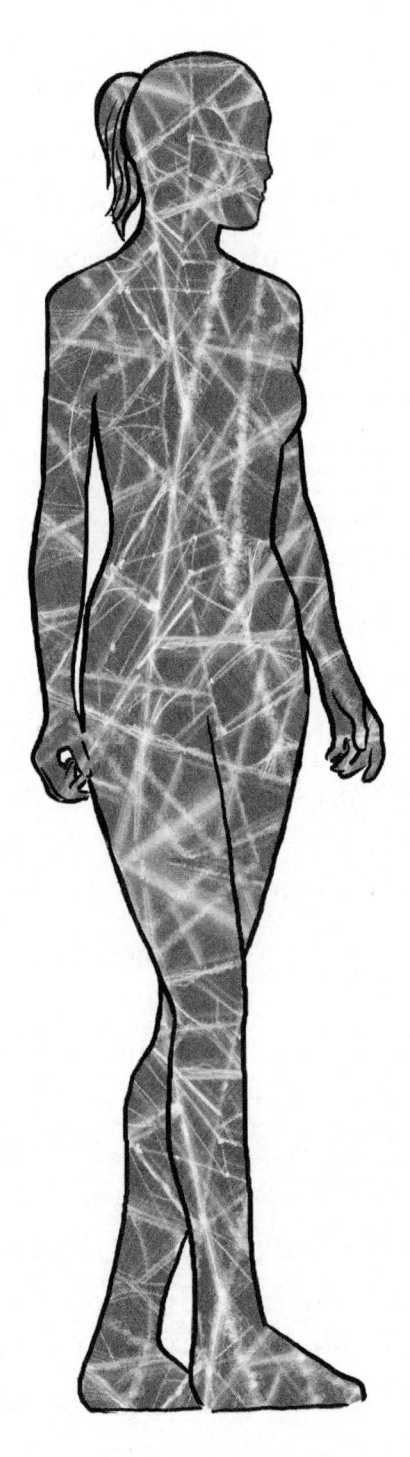

Fascia in the whole body

V – FASCIA AND MOVEMENT

As I have been presenting, the human movement model that many people follow is outdated. The idea of your body as aligned, stacked-up bricks is inaccurate. The image of a little person in your head directing a lever system with pulleys is more like a Disney cartoon and does not fit our mammalian evolution. Moving with the maxim "no pain, no gain" is certainly a thing of the past. What animal would inflict pain on itself? For what? Bigger muscles? Excess muscle tension has not been proven to lead to health.

Movement is the three-dimensional fascial network of posture in action. Myofascial white fibers and muscular red fibers pull in toward the body's core while organizing around strong bones that resist the compression. The skeletal system is organized, balanced, and suspended within the fascial web. As the fascial tissue has elastic properties, it stores energy and gives it back to move with.

For movement, we have the uncontestable, irreducible fact that we have a body this time around, however challenged, and that is how we move through life. How we use it, inhabit it, and move it for health and wellbeing has been a question for me for a long time.

We are biological beings who have always moved to survive: to get food, to work, to chop wood or carry water. But now, our worldly environment doesn't require us to move so much. Food is delivered, often prepared, cars drive themselves, and computers keep us glued to a screen for hours on end. Not much physical activity anymore. What about children? Do they still play outside enough and run around? How do we educate our young ones to move?

Physical training and so-called biomechanical concepts have to change. Hard big muscles might be strong, but they often eliminate flow. Many old-style exercises train the surface muscles such as the vertical abdominals. But you want to access the deeper muscles that are diagonal or spiraling in nature. The typical gym workout trains the body as a machine, which it is not. Much of the old-style muscular repetitive calisthenics such as sit-ups or push-ups are not ideal for training our fascial or biotensegrity systems. In the foreseeable future, we will be leaving the jobs with repetitive movement to the robots. We need authentic or original movement that comes from an inner awareness of our needs, our structure, and our moment-to-moment subtle and energetic changes. The EXploracises are tailored to fit this combination.

Given that part of what I teach is movement education, I am often asked, "Should I swim or do Pilates, or cycle, or lift weights?" Surprising as it may seem, I give everyone the same answer. It is not what you do, but how you do it. The concept of "use" means how you use yourself to do something or what you are doing with yourself as you do any activity. When we look at human development and potential, we generally look at heredity, genetics, and environment. But what about "use"—how you use yourself to do whatever you do?

V – FASCIA AND MOVEMENT

If you ask 10 people to walk across the room, they will all walk in a different way. Yet each style will get you there. The principle of "use" is not about how one specific part of the body moves because body parts do not move independently of one another; the whole self is involved, the synchronized embodiment. Use is an orchestrated activity of your whole self. USE for us humans includes our biological evolutionary history and our biographical personal history and our relationship to the planet.

EX – Biographical Personal Use

1. Think about your own history of how you have used yourself according to your environment.
2. How did you sit at the dinner table?
3. Did you have a dinner table? Or dinner at all?
4. How did you walk to school?
5. How did you sit if you were shamed?
6. How did you play after school?
7. As you stand, notice how comfortable you are. Do you stand with ease or effort? How much effort? Are you shifting hip to hip? Are you pulling yourself up, or maybe kind of heaving yourself up? And then dropping back down in a loop? Just note what it feels like, with as little judgment as possible.

EXPLORACISES

Another way to look at use is with the idea of kinesthetic intelligence (KI). We know about intelligence, and these days, we even know about emotional intelligence. But who pays attention to kinesthetic intelligence? *Kine* = to move and *esthesia* = capacity for sensing. Together the words imply *how we sense movement.* KI includes how the body is structured to move. Moving with the larger picture of unity can be very healing when understood properly. We see that movement can elevate our mood, energize our being, or heal traumatic injuries. If we are alive, there is some movement somewhere.

You can see that how you move affects your health. The therapeutic implications of moving in accord with our inner organization or structure are vast, varied, and almost miraculous. Our bodies grow based on how we use them. If we are chronically tensing due to posture, work, or emotions, the tension is distributed globally and, over time, grows into our physicality. Any added pressure or imbalance grows into the connective system and reduces its ability to slide and glide. The potential for our system to manage forces efficiently becomes limited, and the risk of injury increases.

We want to restore dynamic balance because the body responds to demand. The demand can be from mental, physical, emotional, or spiritual sources. Over time, the fascia will create a running body, a sad body, an anxious body, or a joyful body. We know about neuroplasticity in the nervous system, but we also have tissue plasticity in the fascial system. The tissue can learn to lengthen and stay. Bones float in balanced fascial pulls.

Taking this idea even deeper, the forces that you generate create either space or constriction. Much research has been done on the chemical, biochemical, and genetic behaviors of cells and other parts of the body, but these are very often secondary responses to forces in your body. If forces, stresses, pushes, or pulls are localized and maintained in your body, anywhere, then the cells and body chemistry are changed by these forces, and your body adapts and physically changes. This is how many illnesses are created—from minor strains and sprains to disease such as cancers. Cancer cells have been shown to develop from physical forces applied to them.[3]

You have the ability to fundamentally shape your own body, at every level, through how you go about things. That includes the ability to both avoid discomfort and disease, and to actively reverse it or significantly mitigate it once it's there. Awareness of universal forces can have a tremendous influence on this process.

EX – Ground Reaction Force (GRF)

There is a concept in physics called the *ground reaction force.*

1. You can stand on the Earth in a balanced way, so that the total or net force on you is zero.
2. Your weight acting downward is exactly balanced by the Earth's energy pushing back up on you.
3. You need absolutely no effort to be upright because the Earth is always there, balancing your weight pushing down with exactly the same force pushing up.
4. Try it, or imagine it.
5. It may be easier to feel when running—that spring back up that you get from the ground. Think kangaroo.

EXPLORACISES

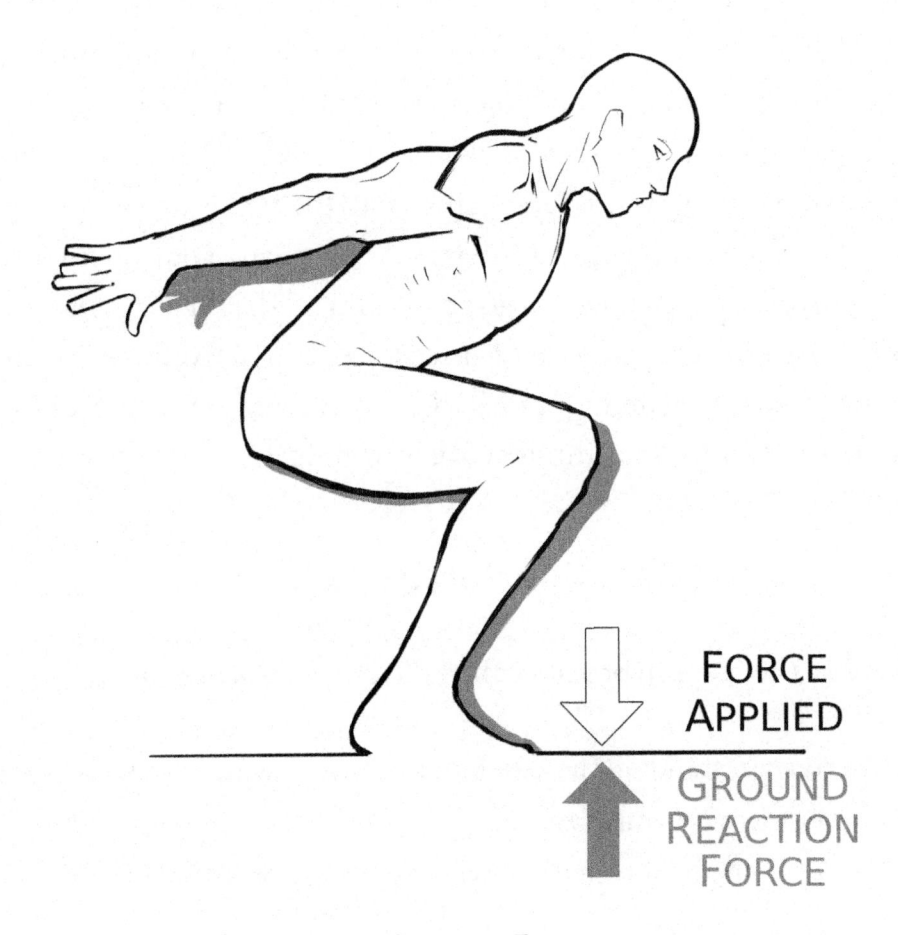

Ground Reaction Force

You can see after doing this GRF EX that the shift from a compression-based, mechanistic model of the body to a tensionally balanced, realistic model is quite radical. It moves us away from the parts-based perspective of the whole being equal to the sum of the parts toward a systems-based perspective of the whole being greater than the sum of the parts. Fascial biotensegrity support unifies our system into a seamlessly organized dynamic whole where every part is involved in all functions, movement, and being, at all times.

VI – PANDICULATION

A type of movement that specifically demonstrates unity and moves the whole body is called *pandiculation.* It is the involuntary stimulation of the soft tissues. You most commonly see (and feel) it in humans and animals waking up from sleeping, naturally doing what looks like "stretching." It may look like a stretch, but when we pandiculate, we're actually contracting muscles that have been inactive. It is our innate response to the sensations of lack of movement and to the pressure that has built up in our muscles. It is our nervous system's natural way of waking up our sensorimotor system and preparing us for movement. We and other vertebrates tend to automatically pandiculate when we have not moved for a while. You have seen a cat or dog arch their back, or a baby reach their arms up, upon waking.

Pandiculation sends biofeedback to our nervous system, expressing the level of contraction in our muscles. This helps to prevent the buildup of chronic muscular stress, allowing the gamma nervous system that regulates our level of tension to reset, reducing muscular tension and inviting voluntary control.

Thomas Hanna, the founder of Clinical Somatic Education, saw the pain and limited movement prevalent in modern society and believed that pandiculation could help. He developed a type of exercise that incorporates pandiculation. He taught eccentric contraction—that is, muscles are lengthening while they are voluntarily engaged.

As I have mentioned, with neuroscience we know that the human brain, as well as the nervous and fascial systems, can change—this is *plasticity*. If we can learn to constrict, we can learn to stop the constriction. Hanna's work is effective because it's an extension of our innate neuromuscular functioning. The technique of voluntary pandiculation allows us to reset the fascial system and reduce our resting level of muscles, while finding more ease in both stillness and movement.[4]

EX – Pandiculation

1. Next time you wake up, pause.
2. Become aware of the tightness in your muscular and fascial systems.
3. Allow these systems to begin to move and pandiculate. It may feel like stretching.
4. Notice how you feel after.

VI – PANDICULATION

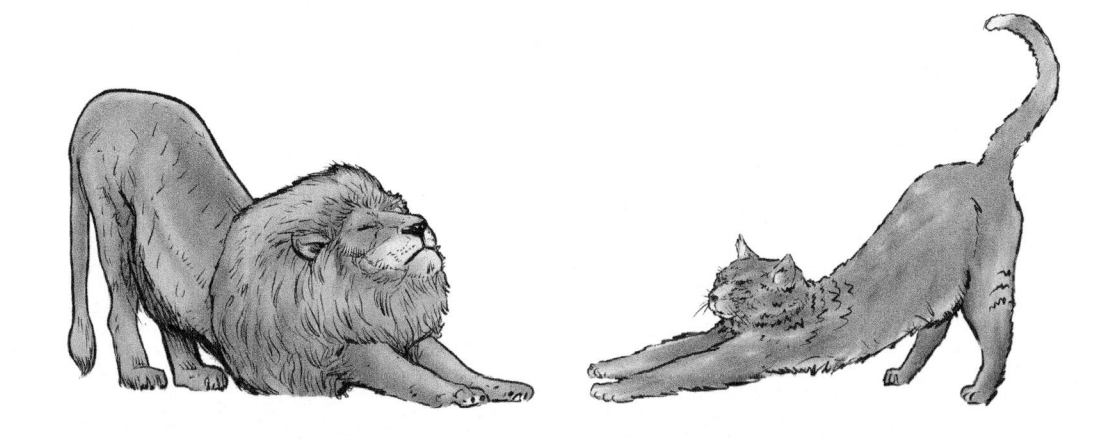

Pandiculation

CHAPTER 2

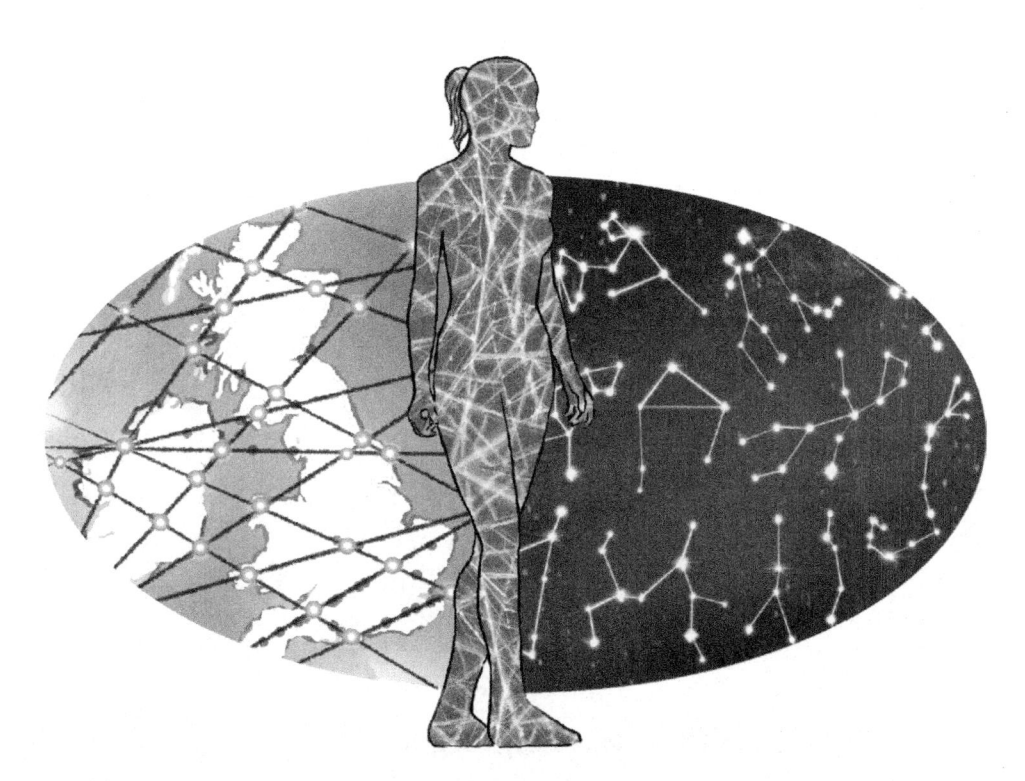

HEAVEN AND EARTH MEET IN SYNCHRONIZED EMBODIMENT

I – UNIVERSAL LAWS OF PHYSICALITY

Synchronized embodiment includes the relationship of our physical, mental, emotional, and spiritual body to the Earth and the other heavenly bodies. There is universality in the bodily functions. We all breathe air that comes to us from above. We all are in contact with the same planet that comes to us from below. We all have a healthy range for blood pressure, heart rate, temperature, body weight, etc. All our knees bend one way and not another. Digestion goes down, not up. Our nervous system cannot operate at high activation for a long time. We have a comfortable resting length for muscles and our fascial structure. We have synchronization within us and around us to our near and far environment.

Our body re–members. The members or parts get put together from information within and around us. Our bodies hold, cherish, hide, or display every experience or encounter we have had, every time and place we have been—all live in the fabric of our body and being. Layers of meaning are woven into our muscles, and memories are etched into our bones. Stories are imprinted on our fascia, and deep feelings of grief or joy pierce our hearts. Breath touches it all, including what is on the surface and what is deep inside.

Many people talk about the body but really have no idea how the body best functions. I find it noteworthy that there is such a split between mind and body that you can go to a university and get a degree in some kind of body-related therapy or work and never have any connection whatsoever to your own body, or anyone else's for that matter.

Years ago, I had a woman approach me. She was getting her PhD in the Alexander Technique. And she called me and said she was thinking about having hands-on sessions. I said to her, "You are getting a PhD in a somatic or body-related discipline, and you have never had the experience of what that bodily sensation is?" She said, "That's right." And she never came for a session, and she got her degree. Understand that the Alexander Technique involves both sides of the brain—the cognitive left side and the experiential right side. She was missing half of the information.

Another example of this: I have attended conferences and heard people who are "experts" in their somatically related field say something like "pull your shoulders back" to a group of thousands. This idiom or directive is so detrimental. Try it for a moment. Pull your shoulders back. How comfortable is it? How long do you stay there? Does your body want to do this? Of course, we all know the answer is no. And yet popular culture continues to prescribe and advise people all the time to pull their shoulders back. I have other ideas about how to solve the issue or problem of why somebody would need to be told to pull their shoulders back.

EXPLORACISES

EX – Synchronized Embodiment and Non-doing

1. The reason you are told to pull your shoulders back is because your shoulders were drooping forward.
2. To droop them forward you need to be pulling the muscles on the front of your upper torso. You need to be contracting them and pulling them in and down in front. Try it.
3. Now when somebody sees the drop, they will tell you to pull your shoulders back.
4. And you may do that. But notice that you have never changed the forward and down pull in your upper chest or torso.
5. So now you are pulling the shoulders forward and pulling them back at the same time.
6. No wonder you are confused and your body says no—let alone how this restricts your breathing.

So now let's try something else.

1. Become aware of the pull forward and down in your shoulders in relationship to your whole self. Feel what your version of this "shoulder drooping" might be.
2. Does one side pull more than the other side?
3. Is the pull low near your armpit, or is it high in your shoulder?
4. Notice the pull. How does it affect your whole tensegrity, your fascial self?
5. Begin to wonder about the emotions related to the pull. Is it a defensive pull? Or a protective pull? A pull to protect a wounded heart?

I – UNIVERSAL LAWS OF PHYSICALITY

6. And what emotions go along with this? Are you afraid and defending out of fear? Or are you sad and protecting yourself from being wounded again?
7. What happens as you notice these patterns? Is there any change in the pull? Did your breathing change if the pull lessened?
8. As the pulls decrease, notice that your shoulders are less drooped forward.
9. Now you can consciously allow your shoulders to widen. It is true that your shoulders were forward before, and now they are more back. But how you got there is very different from directly pulling them back.
10. Often, there are deeper explorations to be done to sort out the need to pull one's shoulders forward in the first place, as your whole body, mind, and spirit are part of that pattern.
11. This synchronized embodiment process gives you the opportunity to see the total pattern of your experience of yourself and to do something about it. Something lasting.
12. I deeply believe that part of why this works is that we are built for wellbeing, so just bringing your attention to the holding will start a shift.

It is also possible to have synchronized embodiment with another. I was reading to my two-year-old grandson as he sat on my lap. He was enjoying the story and moving and squirming in delight as he listened. I supported every bit of him as he moved. He wiggled, and his body was constantly adjusting to his thinking, listening, and emotional state. And I supported him wherever he was. I shifted my attention and my bodily position as he moved, to be sure I supported his every adjustment. No words were spoken about this, but it was palpable to both of us. Most of us did not get this support or attunement, but the circuits are still there. They did not get activated back then, but they can be activated now. Circuits can reconnect for moment-to-moment support.

EX – Synchronized Embodiment and Movement

1. Stand in a comfortable position. Feel your weight contacting the ground.
2. Slowly begin to shift your weight from one foot to the other foot.
3. As you do, at every spot along the way, feel your weight pushing into the ground, and the support coming up to meet that exact weight (GRF).
4. Renew in every moment: Heaven coming down and Earth going up, creating your synchronized embodiment.

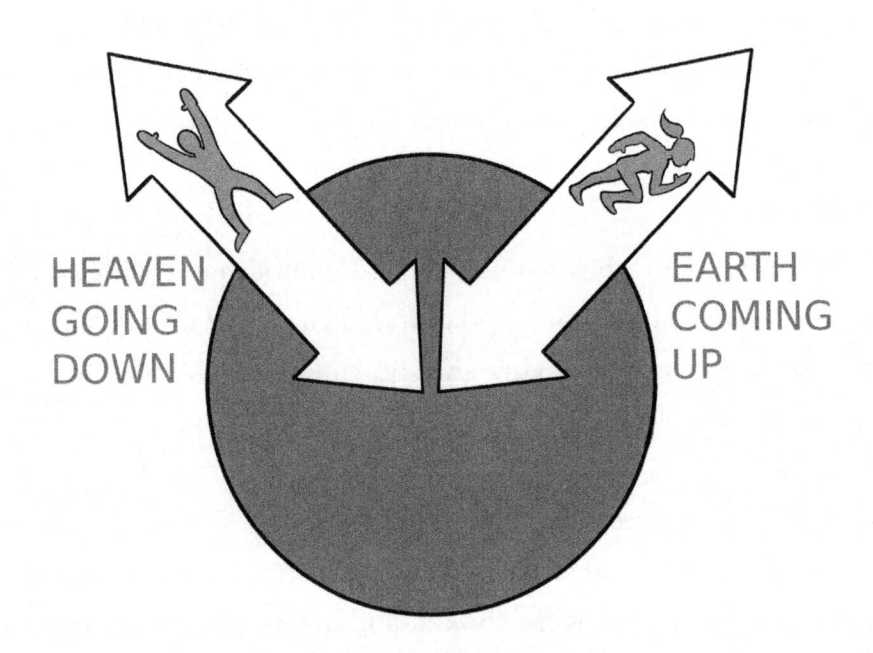

II – COHERENCE

Another word for what I am talking about is somatic *coherence.* The idea is important as we look at our patterns of embodiment to help us manage life, in our surroundings, and with each other. Coherence is a state of equilibrium, homeostasis, and peace of mind. It is both solid and down to Earth, and at the same time ethereal and heavenly. Heaven and Earth meet in synchronized embodiment. Our earthly bodies float in the divine with coherence.

> "When a complex system is far from equilibrium, small islands of coherence, in a sea of chaos, have the capacity to shift the entire system to a higher order."
>
> —*Ilya Prigogine*

With our own overwhelm or watching someone else, we can see that our systems get fragmented or kind of fly apart. It can feel like a pinball machine, balls bouncing all over, as we get overwhelmed or anxious. This can happen with both pleasure or difficulty. Energy is bouncing all over. When this happens to us, we get discombobulated and lose the coherence and organization of the system, and we are not able to direct our physicality toward health. Our embodiment is not synchronized. As you read this next paragraph, feel your somatic interpretation of it inside yourself.

A scientist who studied insects wanted to study fireflies, so he went to Malaysia. He settled into his bungalow, and when darkness fell, he took a big glass jar and went to the river and caught a bunch of fireflies. He brought them back to his bungalow and closed the windows and let them out. At first, they flew all around and lit up randomly at different times (like the pinball machine). Soon he saw that two, close together, began pulsing together. Then two more on the other side of the room also flashed together. Before long, there were islands of unified pulsing, synchronized rhythm. The fireflies inside began to resonate with each other. Eventually, the whole room was flashing as one light.

All the systems in our human body are meant to pulse together, to energize in harmony with each other. Success is when they communicate together, and they are flexible and adaptive to the environment in the present moment. I don't know what fireflies do to be present, but they need some kind of presence to pulse or vibrate together.

II – COHERENCE

EX – Coherence

1. How does this translate for you as you read it?
2. Notice if your own energy is bouncing all around randomly like the fireflies when first released.
3. You may feel it as anxiety or fear or overwhelm.
4. The first response we all have is to not feel it or to get rid of it.
5. With that we leave our body behind and go to our head.
6. Instead, feel the movement and then begin to consciously move the bouncing particles to bounce together one by one.
7. Picture the fireflies and you can begin to coordinate and pulse your own system together, in this present moment.
8. The here and now is the organism functioning well with biological systems pulsing together—brain, body, emotions, and spirit, flexible and organized. When this is not happening, we are oriented to another moment, a moment of some kind of intensity or overwhelm, as trauma is a disorder in the ability to be in the here and now.

Developing the capacity to anchor in somatic coherence is a practice, as we tend to lose and regain coherence with the ups and downs of life. The EXploracises offer different methods and degrees of difficulty for you to establish a new take on how you perceive your reality. The possibilities include feeling more energetic, a greater sense of wellbeing, and more excitement to move into the life you authentically want. Each of us individually contributes to the evolving of the species. We are moving away from a mechanistic, hierarchical world to an intuitive, coherently informed society. This is a new type of evolution for us. For this we must include the universal forces.

EXPLORACISES

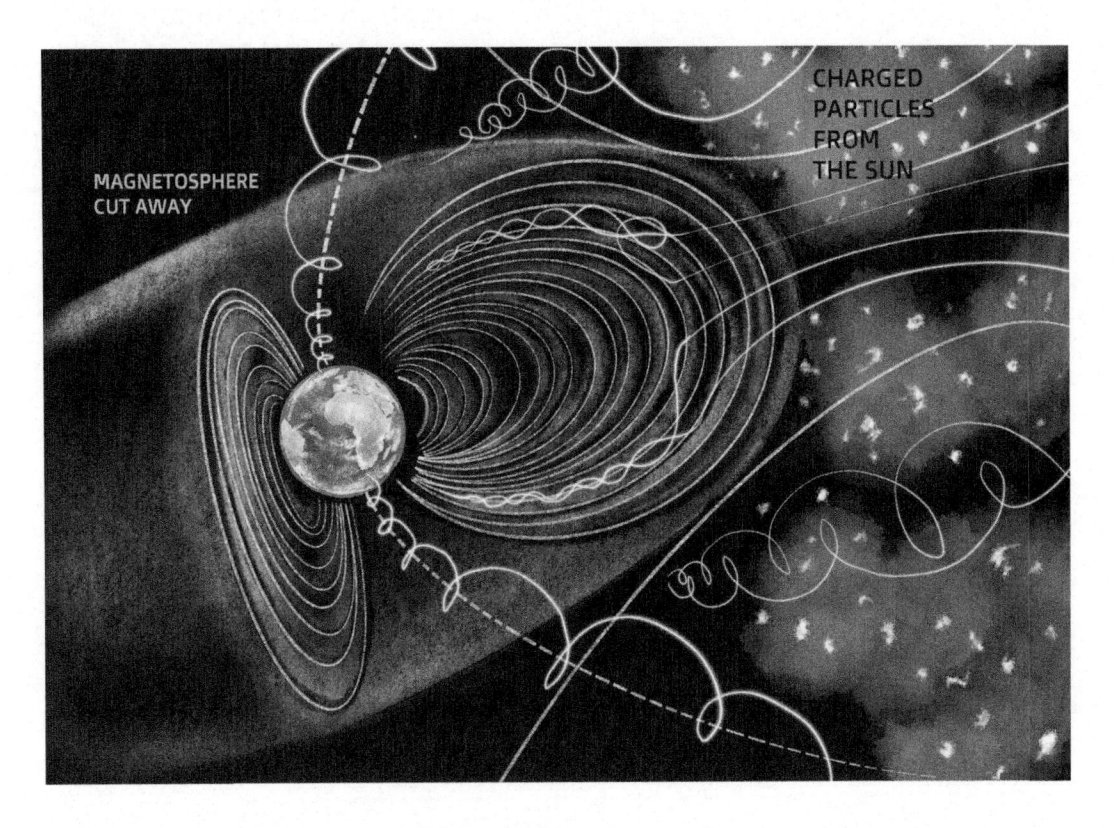

Magnetosphere cut away

III – UNIVERSAL FORCES FROM HEAVEN AND EARTH

The Heavens meet the Earth. The Earth is alive and vibrant and changing and moving all the time. The Earth gives us our food, our minerals, our trees, sustenance for daily life. The center is made of metals that affect the energy on the surface. The work of Rory Duff, geobiologist (one who studies how the Earth affects life), tells us there is a whole system of ley lines, mapped out on the Earth's surface with different kinds or degrees of energy.[1] Some locations have more energy than others. These are often the sites of healing centers or traditional religious or spiritual places of worship. Why do some people feel comfortable in one location, but not another?

EXPLORACISES

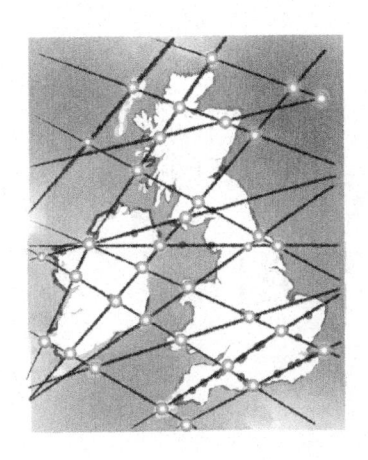

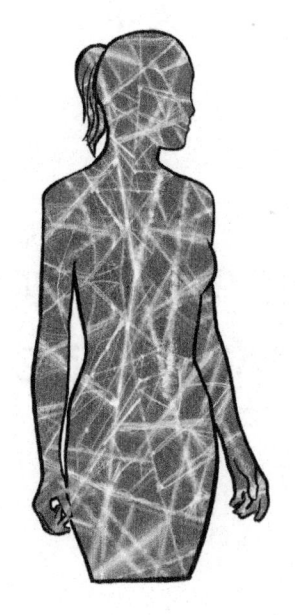

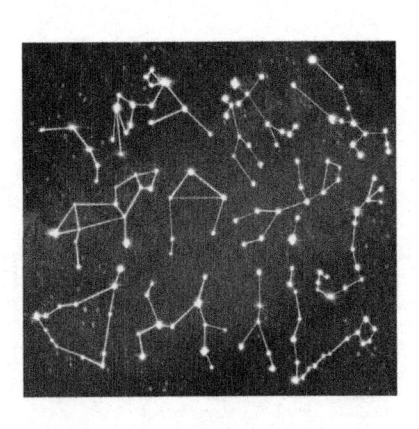

Heaven and Earth meet: ley lines, fascia, and cosmos

The Earth meets the Heavens. The Heavens (or cosmos) contain our surrounding planets, giving us light from the sun and energies from the near and far, small and large planets. Solar rays light our days, warming our Earth and our bodies. The moon lights our way by night and moves the tides, touching the water inside us with deep emotions. The sky, filled with air that we breathe, fills us with life-giving oxygen.

Heaven and Earth meet in synchronized embodiment. With gravity, the Heavens and the Earth are attracted to each other. It is simply a pull between two objects. As you stand on the Earth, you are affected by both forces. You could say that we pay attention to gravity like a fish pays attention to water. We don't consciously pay attention to it, but our biological system sorts it out for us and is evolved to use it to our advantage. But many people blame gravity for their slumped posture. In reality, if you were floating in space with no gravity, you would not be upright at all. Gravity gives us our upright posture, if we

III – UNIVERSAL FORCES FROM HEAVEN AND EARTH

allow it to. Slumped posture has more to do with our internal state. Ida Rolf, creator of the popular massage style known as Rolfing, said it well: "Gravity is the therapist."[2]

She is saying: The movement of gravity shows us where we pull down and tighten. These pulls can be caused by many emotional, social, and/or environmental factors, but understanding antigravity, GRF, and support can help to restore balance.

Gravity does not work the way most people think it does. Laws of gravity that most are familiar with are outdated and have been superseded by Einstein's General Theory of Relativity, which in the near future will be seen to be outdated. We are part of the geometry of the universe. Gravity is not a force that drags us down. The surprising fact is that the contact you feel of the ground under your feet or chair is not of you going down, but of that surface accelerating up underneath you to support you. The support coming up is called antigravity (created by the Earth's centrifugal force from spinning), as you read about in the section on ground reaction force (Chapter 1, section V).

In physics—in particular, in biomechanics—related to Newton's Third Law, the ground reaction force (GRF) is the force exerted by the ground on a body in contact with it. When the body is moving, the GRF increases due to acceleration forces. For example, when someone is running, the GRF increases to up to two or three times the body weight. For the scientifically minded: to find the ground reaction force or the magnitude of the acceleration due to gravity, use the following formula. When a person stands still, this ground reaction force is equal to the person's mass multiplied by the gravitational acceleration, which is 9.8 meters per second, squared. Squared means meters per second per second. The floor accelerates into you, at rest on the surface of the Earth. This also means that every second an object is in free fall, gravity will cause the velocity of the object to increase 9.8 m/s. So, after one second, the object is traveling at 9.8 m/s. Ignoring the effects of air resistance, the speed of the object falling freely will increase by about 9.8 meters per second (32 ft/s) every second.

EX – Your Experience of Gravity

1. If you think gravity is a heavy force pushing you toward the ground, and that is all there is, then you will end up pushed down.
2. But if you recognize or know that there is a counterbalancing energy coming up from the Earth, then you can feel supported or even weightless, using gravity to your advantage, to come into upright posture, remembering that posture is a phase of movement, not an end product.

Our posture is constantly recalibrating and reconfiguring. We need to be free enough to allow that to happen. Part of our synchronized embodiment is our wobbly structure. Our joints are not rigid; they are movable, not stable. If we think this is a mistake, and we stiffen our joints to not be wobbly, we cut off information about what is happening at the joints. We are continuously adjusting to our thoughts from inside and to the stimuli from our environment. With the internal organization and postural reflexes transported through us, we are constantly refining support in our movement with small adjustments. Watch a toddler when he or she is learning to walk.

III – UNIVERSAL FORCES FROM HEAVEN AND EARTH

EX – Space between Heaven and Earth

1. Lie down on your back.
2. Become aware of the edges of you meeting open space—above, both sides, top of head, and bottom of feet.
3. Notice what of you is in contact with the ground.
4. Let 2 and 3 meet.
5. Become aware of space between body parts. If your arms are resting on your belly, there is space between your upper and lower arm. Space between fingers and toes. Between your legs.
6. Back to your contact with the ground.
7. Let 5 and 6 meet.
8. As you stay with the space around you, it is possible to mesh with the solid contact. And you can feel more porous in your contact with the Earth, like the soil is aerated.

EX – Nature in You

1. The synchronized embodiment of you includes the five major elements in the natural world. Explore these:
   element – nature – human
2. Wood – tree – bone
3. Water – ocean – fluid
4. Air – breeze – breath
5. Fire – volcano – heat
6. Metal – iron ore – minerals

You have a relationship with the natural world around you. You and the natural world share the elements. She is your terrain, soil, wind, water, and your soul fire. Might that connection be helpful? Native Americans referred to animals and plants as "all my relations" and did not consider them "natural resources" for exploitation (like many modern people do).

EX – Egypt Body

There is great interest now in the ancient civilization of Egypt and the skills they had in building, astronomy, astrology, and more. I am fascinated by their physicality, the bodies of the ancient Egyptians.

1. Look at any image of the pictures drawn on the walls of temples and pyramids.
2. Notice the uprightness. I see no one slumping. Why aren't the researchers interested in this?
3. There was one series of figures that showed the sequence of life. Even the old man was not bent over. He held a cane to depict his age. If it was a modern picture, he would have been slouched over.
4. Find your Egypt body.

Looking at modern civilization, I see so many people collapsed downward, whether from the pressure and emotional stress of life, or they are looking down at their phones or computers. When I look at images of the Egyptians, the word *upright* comes to mind. This poised posture does not seem to be a priority today.

III – UNIVERSAL FORCES FROM HEAVEN AND EARTH

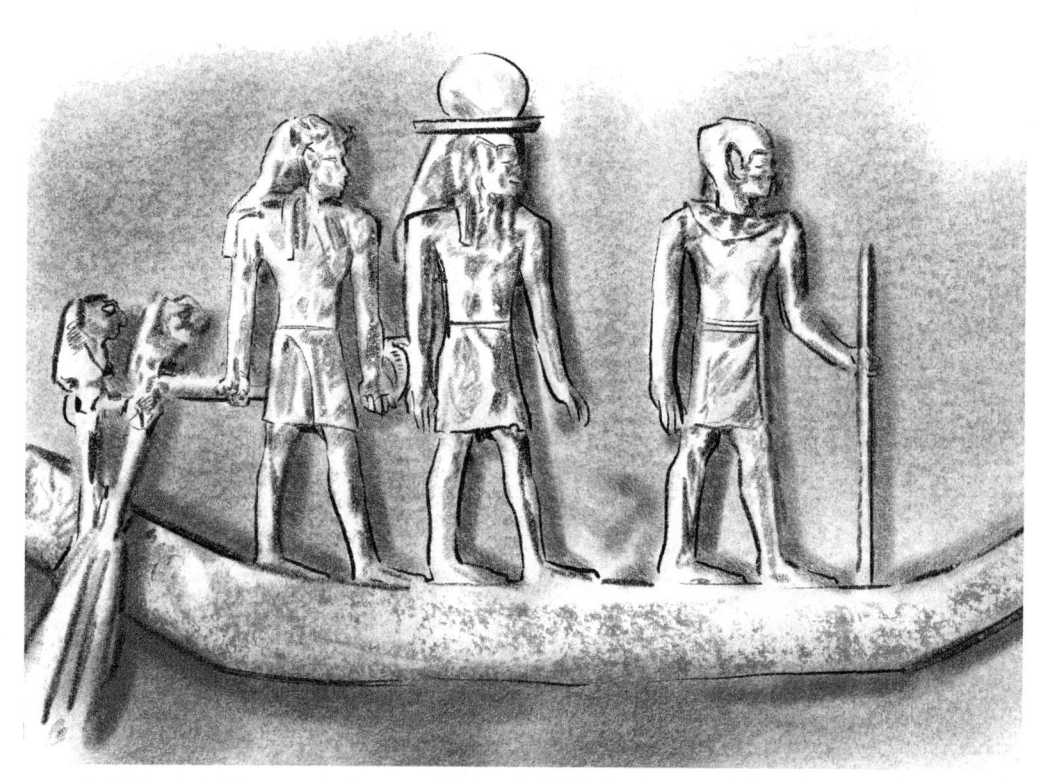

Egypt Body

IV – SPIRALS

Our interior muscles and organs are a whirlwind of spirals, and those spiraling flows of synchronized embodiment extend into the air around us. The connection between Heaven and Earth, and gravity and antigravity, is diagonal curves or spirals. Spirals are the design of our universe. They are everywhere in Heaven and on Earth: the spinning planets, nature, physical bodies, DNA, and our movements. Dr. Stephen Levin says that even our bones bounce in a spiral shape.[3] Some spirals start on the ground, spiral through the body, and continue up to the sky. Some we can see and others we cannot see, but they are there. Sometimes we see one curved line or part of a spiral. An airplane goes in a straight line but ends up in a curved pattern. Spirals often come in pairs: one in one direction and one in another direction. We see this double spiral in many ancient temples, as a symbol of our life patterns. Spirals are often fractals or repeated patterns.

Similarly, our experiences come in spirals. We have layers—like tree rings. Layers of our experience: the past, or not now, affects the now, the present moment. Some scientists say that tree rings

IV – SPIRALS

are spirals, not rings, not two-dimensional, but three-dimensional.[4] Rings are spirals of experience. The spirals are like a hose or tube—experience and breath flow through them. Sometimes there is a kink in the hose, a blockage, a "wrong" turn off the path. We want to get the spiral channel flowing again. We have so many spiral channels and tubes inside us—the heart, intestines, ears, and digestive system are a few examples. Begin to think about and feel the spiral muscles, tubes, and pulls inside you. The spirals can connect parts of you, conscious me and unconscious me. Every journey is a spiral.

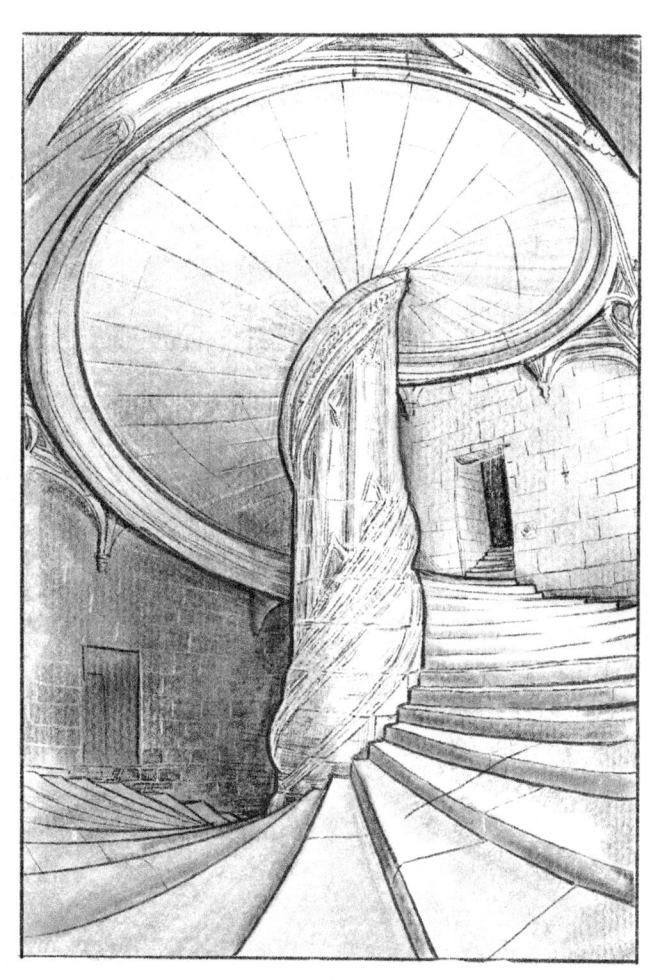

The Da Vinci Spirals

EX – Foot Spirals

1. Draw a diagonal line with your finger on the top of your foot, from the big toe to the outer heel. Do the right foot, then the left.
2. Draw a diagonal line from the pinky toe to the inner heel. On the right foot, then the left.
3. Do the lines feel even, muscularly and energetically?
4. These diagonal lines are the beginning of the spiral lines going up your body that you will discover in the next few EX.

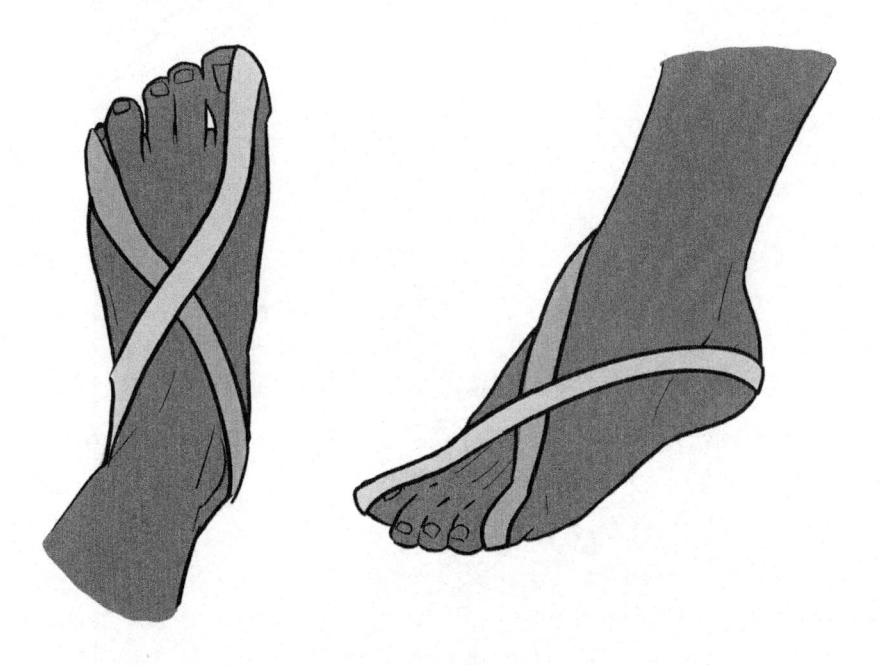

Foot Spirals

IV – SPIRALS

EX – Spiral Arm Hug

1. In a standing position, rock forward and backward, on your toes, then heels. Be aware of your support. Rock less forward, and less back. Keep lessening your forward and back until you come center. As you come center, it is possible to feel the upthrust from the ground into your foot spirals, in the upward direction. It is alchemy—two things produce a third new thing. Decreasing forward-and-back motion reveals up.
2. Shift from foot to foot with straight legs, as it stimulates the baroreceptors, which are the blood pressure feedback loops.
3. Begin to bend your knees as you shift. Let your body sway, breathe. Let your head tilt, as you are spiraling from side to side.
4. Add letting your arms swing around your body. Feel the suspension or floating quality as you travel from side to side. Swinging is a wonderful rhythmic movement that we mammals have done for millions of years.
5. Engage your spirals into a body hug. Each time you get to a side, pause for a moment in the hug. Let yourself feel the power of your own hug. Perhaps remembering, *nobody held me, nobody listened to me.* Hold and listen now.
6. Let the movement come to less and then none.

Feel the result of what you have done. Notice the changes. Any less freeze? Any openings? Be open to learn a new process or gain a fresh understanding about yourself. Bring the openings to the next thing you do.

EXPLORACISES

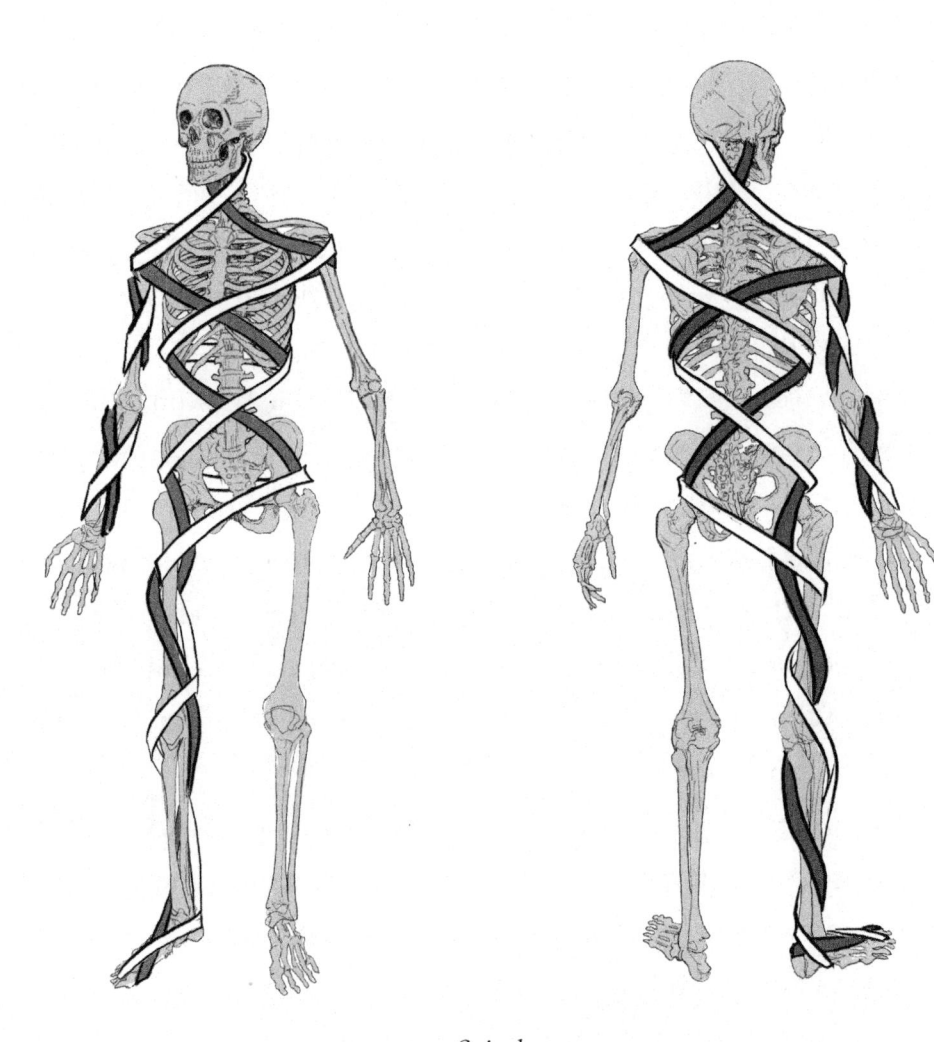

Spirals

IV – SPIRALS

EX – Walking with Spirals

This can be initiated lying on the floor or done as a simpler version as you sit in a chair. Two inches below your navel is your *dan tian,* or *hara,* the energy center of vitality, also called the *second sacral chakra*. I am calling it "belly" for simplicity, but I don't mean the stomach. This center is used to initiate spirals.

1. Allow your belly to sink to the floor or to your lower back on your exhale. Repeat this step before every movement. Move on the exhale.
2. Repeat step 1. Then bring left knee to belly. Release. Repeat with right knee.
3. Repeat step 1. Then bring right elbow to left bent knee. Release. Repeat with left elbow and right bent knee.
4. Repeat step 1. Then repeat 3 and add head turning with arm movement.
5. Keep right elbow touching left knee, head turned.
6. Straighten left leg and right arm together. Release. Repeat step 5 with right leg and left arm. Straighten right leg and left arm.
7. Stand and take it into walking.
8. Right knee goes forward. And right elbow pulls back. Then left knee goes forward and left elbow pulls back. Feel the spiral twist as you walk.

EXPLORACISES

EX – Spirals of Experience

1. Find an area that seems overly constricted on one side of your body (right shoulder).
2. Then find an area that seems less constricted on the opposite side of your body (left foot).
3. Draw or make a diagonal spiral connection between the two. Spiral the energy from one to the other in a loop around your body.
4. Often, they are over- and under-active parts. No part is activated alone. It is always in relationship to a non-activated part. The activated layer just speaks or screams louder! But it may not be the real problem.
5. After you have done that for two minutes, do the opposite spiral (from your left shoulder to your right foot).
6. Do them both together.

EX – Spiral Twists

1. Notice if you lean or spiral to one side. Or notice if you are crooked in some way.
2. Instead of trying to get rid of the twists, you want to strengthen the opposite spiral.
3. Do the twist to the side that you like to twist to, and go as far as you can go.
4. Find the elasticity or springy spot, and then spring back to center. Do that a few times.

IV – SPIRALS

5. Then let yourself spring beyond center, to the side you don't like to go to.
6. Go as far as you can to that side in that spiral and bounce back to the other side. Be sure to include your head in the spiral.
7. Keep going side to side.
8. The double-helix spiral is used as the DNA symbol and in the caduceus, the medical insignia of two intertwined snakes.

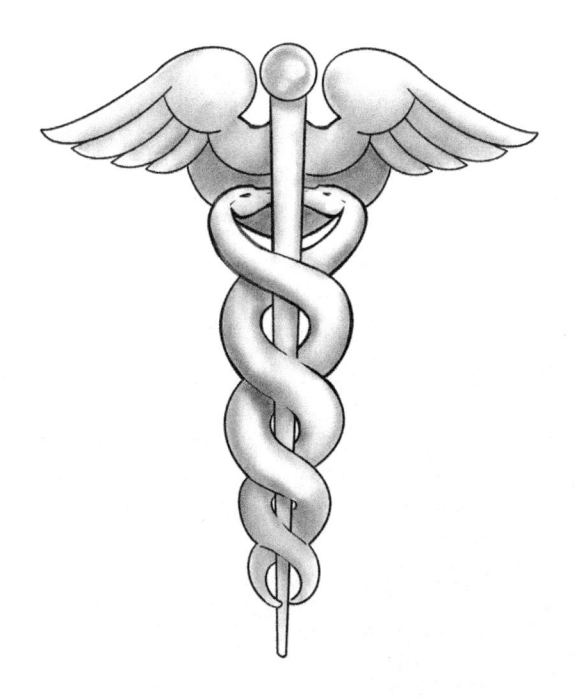

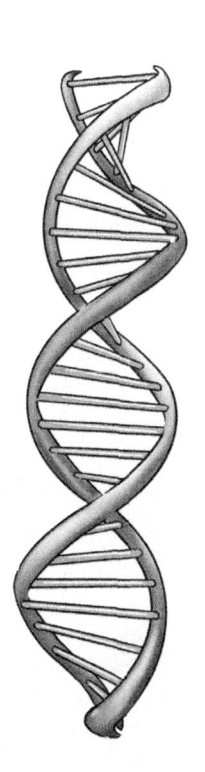

Double-helix Spiral

EX – Turtle Spirals

1. Lie on the floor face down with large pillows under your belly.
2. Swim or move like a turtle and feel if one side is stronger than the other, spiraling from right arm forward, then left leg forward.
3. Then left arm and right leg.
4. You can also do this lying on your back, reaching one arm forward, then the other, while your legs are responding.

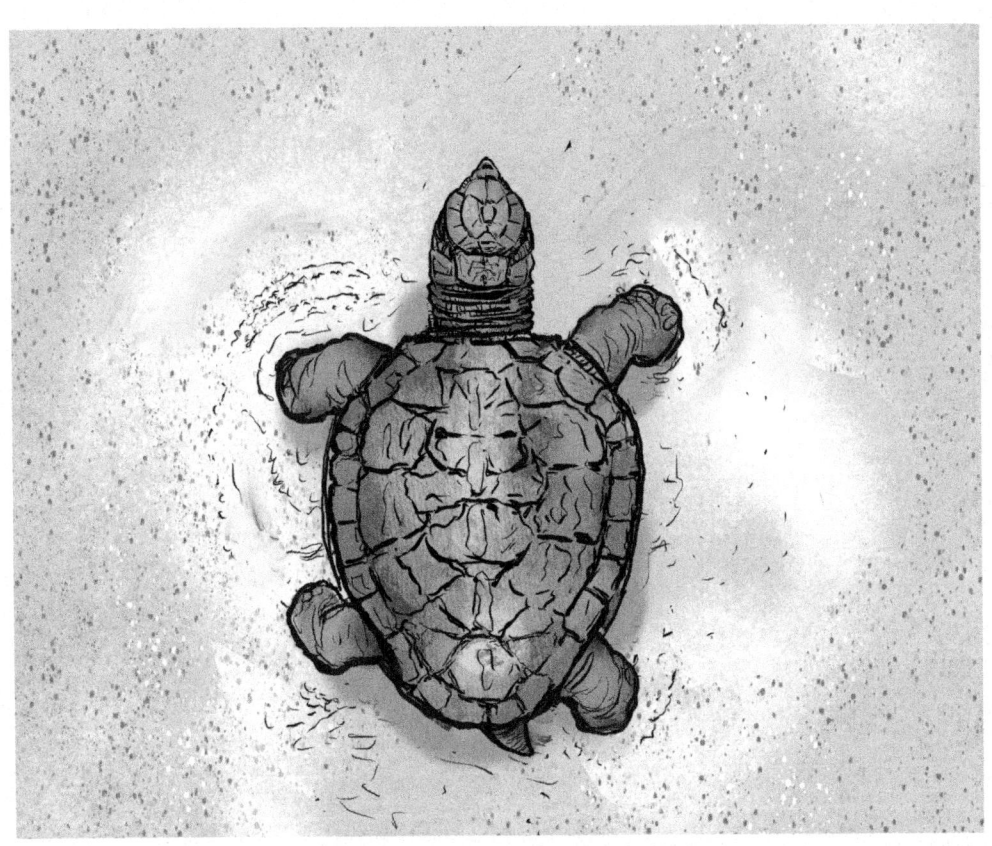

Turtle demonstrating cross pattern spiral

V – Being in the PRESENT MOMENT or Having PRESENCE

Synchronized embodiment has an element of the present moment, which is the moment you are in, whether you consciously choose it or not. *Trying* to be in the present moment, or even being aware of being in the present moment, is different from being present. Trying to be present has obvious implications of effort and doing. Trying also implies that you are not satisfied with where you are, and you want to be somewhere else, like the present. Yet, if you are daydreaming while crossing the street, it will be helpful to come back to the present moment. Awareness of being in the present moment has less doing and less efforting but still implies that there is a me watching another me being present.

EXPLORACISES

EX – Ways to Think About the Present Moment

1. Allow awareness to come to you of your inner and outer environment: the color of the walls, the shapes, the sensory experiences, and related bodily sensations.
2. Touch the first expression of goodness.
3. When you are walking in the woods, enjoying the trees and Earth below your feet, you are in the present moment without thinking that you are present.

Actually, being present just is. You don't say you are present, but someone else might notice it. We might say that this person has a kind of presence. The person with the presence is usually not trying to do anything or be anything. Yet being in the present moment is often interpreted as a goal or an effort. Lack of presence is dissociation—an attraction to lack of presence of self.

When you decide to try to be present, you are dividing your attention by asking your mind to put attention on your sensory environment and negotiating your experience from your mind *and* body. You are still having the separate you perceive something. Yet when you are walking in the woods, enjoying your surroundings, you are seamlessly belonging to a moment, without the dual perspective. So, trying to be present implies a divide. In the firefly story, we recognize that the fireflies had to have some kind of presence to light up together. What is that subtle level of presence where there is no efforting, yet you are not in a daydream? I call that synchronized embodiment of Heaven and Earth.

V – BEING IN THE PRESENT MOMENT

This story depicts it well. I found it in a book called *The Elegance of the Hedgehog* by Muriel Barbery, and it describes a New Zealand Māori ritual dance.

> Then when the New Zealand players began their haka, I got it. In their midst was this very tall Māori player, really young. I'd had my eye on him right from the start, probably because of his height to begin with but then because of the way he was moving. A really odd sort of movement, very fluid but above all very focused, I mean very focused within himself. Most people, when they move, well, they just move depending on whatever's around them...
>
> Either you move and you're no longer whole, or you're whole and you can't move. But that player, when I saw him go out onto the field, I could tell there was something different about him. I got the impression that he was moving, yes, but by staying in one place. Crazy, no? When the haka began, I concentrated on him. It was obvious he wasn't like the others...
>
> Everyone was enthralled by him, but no one seemed to know why. Yet it became obvious in the haka: he was moving and making the same gestures as the other players (slapping the palms of his hands on his thighs, rhythmically drumming his feet on the ground, touching his elbows, and all the while looking the adversary in the eyes like a mad warrior), but while the others' gestures went toward their adversaries and the entire stadium who were watching, this player's gestures stayed inside him, stayed focused upon him, and that gave him an unbelievable presence and intensity... That Māori player

was like a tree, a great indestructible oak with deep roots and a powerful radiance—everyone could feel it. And yet you also got the impression that the great oak could fly, that it would be as quick as the wind, despite, or perhaps because of, its deep roots. …The commentators were sort of hungover, but they couldn't hide the fact that they'd seen something really beautiful: a player who was running without moving, leaving everyone else behind him. And the others, who seemed by comparison to move with frenzied and awkward gestures, were incapable of catching up with him. So I said to myself: There, I have managed to witness motionless movement in the world: is that something worth carrying on for?[5]

CHAPTER 3

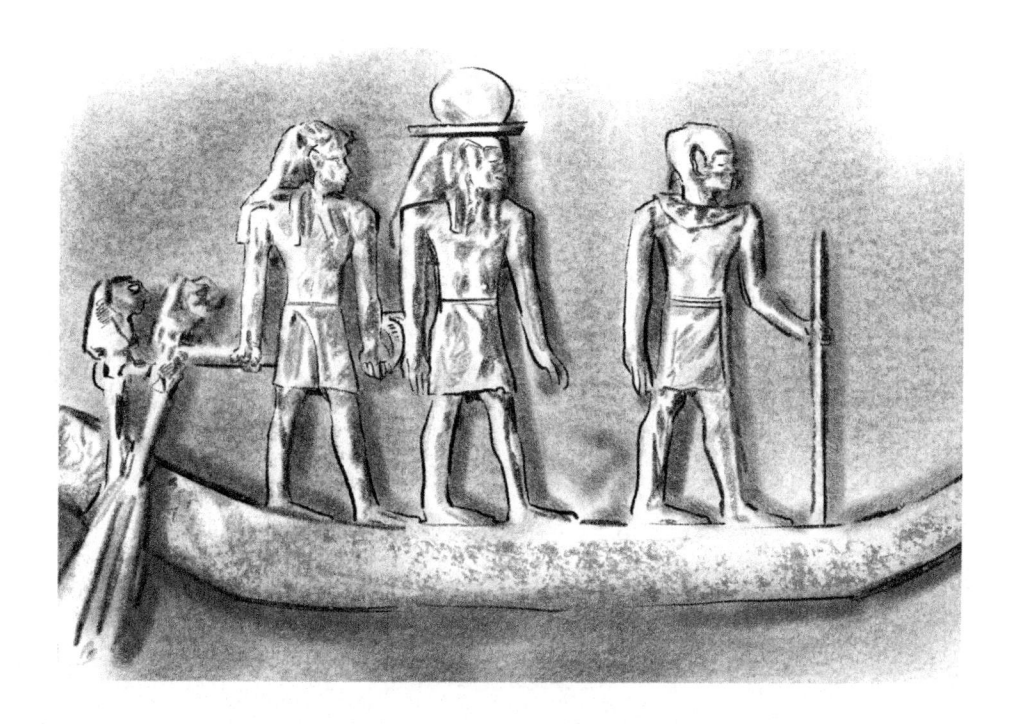

PHYSICALITY

I – INTRODUCTION TO PHYSICALITY

As you have read, we are looking at a new paradigm of physicality. Instead of working out, we are working in. Instead of listening to others, we are listening to our own inner guidance. Instead of a mechanistic, isolated machine model, we are recognizing a tensionally balanced, supported structure, with emotions and sensations, that is connected to his/herself and to others. This requires a body that is made of material that can adapt.

The body's software store: You would need a large shopping cart to purchase all the materials needed to make a body, but connective tissue manages to build all of them—something like strings, elastics, sheets, sacs, insulating material, bone, and springs. Your connective tissue cells make all of these from three simple elements: water, gels, and fibers. The cornea of your eye, the enamel covering your teeth, and the valves of your heart are three of the extraordinary connective tissues arrayed on display and at work in your body.[1]

I – INTRODUCTION TO PHYSICALITY

One very familiar comment that I hear:

Student: I don't feel my body.

But if I continue the inquiry and ask:

Me: Do you feel your glasses on your nose? Do you feel your feet touching the floor? Do you feel your stomach growl sometimes? Etc.
Student: Yes.
Me: Then you feel your body.

Then the next question—

Student: How can I learn to listen to my body?
Me: Start by listening. When you are hungry, eat. Stop when full. When you need to go to the bathroom, go. When you are thirsty, drink. When you are tired, rest. This is "evidence-based."

Said in jest. (Of course, you do not need evidence on this one.)

EX – What Are You Doing in Your Physicality?

1. As you begin to observe your body, there are different ways to see and feel your physicality, or what you are organized to do.
2. Notice tone, restrictions, color changes, temperature, pulse. Notice what you are doing—resting, thinking, planning, (reading!), etc.
3. What is your body saying? I'm tired, I'm hungry, I'm happy, etc.
4. What is the emotion underneath?

EXPLORACISES

5. Is there any disconnection from self or spirit?
6. Are there any repeated patterns? Are you aware of them?
7. How much of your body speaks and expresses?

"You can observe a lot by just watching."

—*Yogi Berra*

EX – Physicality Musings

- When you become acutely aware of any one part of your body, your whole body/being shows up as background. It's almost like looking at an object while at the same time there is peripheral vision showing you the larger picture.
- Why are so many people hunched over forward or slouching? Our front body is soft with so many vulnerable bits exposed. We need protection. This is one way to get it. There are other ways.
- With tightness or constriction, is it skin, fascia, muscle, bone, or viscera?
- Are body and mind really one? What if I listen to my body as much as I listen to my mind's chatter? Why don't people hate their minds like they hate their bodies? Can you "diet your mind" from destructive thoughts, like you diet with foods? Do you take your mind to the gym to get it in the shape you want?
- When you lose touch with a part of your body, it is called sensory motor amnesia. It often shows up as chronically contracted muscles, interfering with movement, breath, and posture.

I – INTRODUCTION TO PHYSICALITY

- It's not about healing the physical body. It's about discovering the need for the symptoms, and then wondering, *Are these behaviors, thoughts, or emotions still necessary?*
- The inner movement of life has a flow and undulation similar to a jellyfish or another underwater creature that moves as a coherent whole.
- Your neck is a powerful connector. Neck muscles attach to the skull, spine, jaw, upper ribs, upper arms. It's the only hub where five bony systems meet.
- To many people, the cosmetic body is most important. Few appreciate how our bodies work and feel, by becoming kinesthetically aware. Even fewer observe or appreciate their energetic body.
- Touch is mutual all the time. The right kind of attuned touch invites amazing possibilities.
- Not about right or wrong. But about doing and not doing.
- The inner body is where you can rest, as you lower your eyelids.
- We want to connect, and survive.
- Any time you make a local physical change or adjustment, you must bring it into the rhythm of the whole body, or it will not last.

EX – Tension

Many people say, "I carry so much tension." I then explain that in my world, tension, when related to the body, is not used as a noun. A noun is a person, place, or thing. Tension is none of them. It is more accurately used as a verb. I suggest that one can say, "I am tensing." That is what is going on, either consciously or subconsciously.

As we look closer, this interchange says so much. *I carry tension* makes tension a thing that I carry. We have the "I" and the "tension." This separates me from myself; it's the ultimate issue (separation) we all deal with, magnified by any traumatic incident. For example: Because my adaptive pattern was developed for me to survive being abandoned by my caregivers, it seems like I am repeating the abandonment pattern by leaving my adaptive self and the separation as part of a healing process. This makes it not so easy to phrase it the new way, which is "I am tensing." The path to freedom and reintegration reveals our past.

1. The adaptive self includes the collection of feelings, the emotional tensegrity made up of the rage, the anger, the sadness, the hurt, the aloneness, etc.—they are all there, a multifaceted structure.
2. Try it out next time you feel constriction. Bring it to consciousness. Say and feel, "I am tensing."
3. You might stop tensing, or you might continue tensing but begin doing it with awareness and choice, so you can modulate it. Feel yourself tense a little, and then less. Not getting rid of it.

EX – Stimulus and Response

The moment between stimulus and response is the moment of choice.

1. Stimulus: You need to send a text.
2. Habitual response: Drop your head and tighten your hands.
3. Notice the pattern and remember that your neck sometimes hurts.
4. Moment of choice.
5. New response: Decide to respond with less tensing.

I – INTRODUCTION TO PHYSICALITY

EX – Perception of Physicality

Words have different interpretations for different people.

1. Up: seamless, flowing "up," or jagged, pulled "up"?
2. Flowing up is support received from the ground, with no effort.
3. Jagged up is anxiously pulling your shoulders up to your ears with effort.
4. Explore the different versions of "up" and notice when your up is connecting Heaven and Earth or when a constriction is disconnecting Heaven and Earth.
5. Productive heavy and lifeless heavy.
6. The former heavy is weighted contact to the ground with space.
7. The latter heavy is lifeless, lack of energy falling into the ground, not allowing space.
8. Use the heaviness to bounce to the ground and come up. Is there any part of the heaviness that bounces?

Our perception of physicality changes. When we have the experience of "working through an issue," we often feel like we have more space inside, or we feel lighter. What is the reality of this? We did not lose weight nor make a measurable change in space inside. But perhaps we have enlivened the molecules of awareness and invited them into consciousness. Now they are not weighing us down with hidden mysteries of our past. The new field of "Spatial Medicine" is arriving.

In ancient Egyptian lore, it is said that at the time of death, we meet the Egyptian Goddess Maat. She has scales, and she weighs your human heart with a feather, and if your heart is heavier than the feather, too heavy, you must return to Earth. The heaviness and spaciousness are related. If you feel heavy, you probably don't feel spacious. Also, this heaviness has nothing to do with actual weight. I worked with ballet dancers in the '80s, and many were thin as a rail but were very pulled down and heavy (when they were not dancing). And the contrast to this is that we have people with much larger bodies, but they are still light and freely moving. If we look in the animal world, we see polar bears ever so lightly jumping across ice patches. The possibility of this concept was explained further in the section on biotensegrity (Chapter 1, section III).

II – SPECIFICS OF PHYSICALITY

This section includes explanations and clarifications of many concepts of physicality. The body wants to be seen and witnessed. We all have many bodies: an animal body, a social body, a divine body, a cultural body, a primitive body, a cosmic body, no body, and more. In a larger picture, we are also including the energetic, subtle, auric, and collective bodies/fields. They all have various expressions. What we do with our physicality speaks volumes about what we are up to.

Ralph Waldo Emerson, American essayist and poet, once quipped: "What you DO speaks so loud that I cannot hear what you say."

EX – Tracking

The process of paying attention to the sensations in your body is called *tracking*. Tracking engages the felt sense, or the ability to feel sensations, inside your body. Learning to track is step one in beginning to understand and feel your physicality. If you live with your awareness mostly in your head, like many people do, and are not used to paying attention to your body, you may find tracking difficult at first.

As you pay attention to your body, you might say that you don't feel anything (which is also a feeling). But as you continue to pay attention, you may start to notice large things, like weight changes or temperature changes, and eventually, you notice other small movements like buzzy, shaky, wobbly, trembly, tingly, bubbly. This process of tracking sensations can be helpful when overwhelming feelings of fear or anxiety arise.

Sensations you may notice:
queasy, heavy, fluid, dizzy, spacey, tight, achy, frozen, suffocating, contracted, tremulous, disconnected, sweaty, hollow, icy, constricted, expansive, buzzy, shaky, wobbly, hot, trembly, full, numb, tingly, expanded, nervous, floating, electric, wooden, congested, twitchy, bubbly, itchy, calm, energized, smooth, warm, light, cold, streaming, restless, dense, thick, fluttery, flowing, breathless, knotted.

II – SPECIFICS OF PHYSICALITY

EX – Tracking Practice

Eyes open or closed. You will be putting your hand on different parts of your body and noticing any sensations: flow or holding or changes? In this tracking EX, we are trying to find differences. (When I first put my hand here, I felt nothing; now I feel warmth.) There is no right or wrong way to do it.

1. Place your hand on the back of your head where your skull meets your neck, two fingers on your skull and two fingers on your neck. You are touching the reptilian brain where survival lives.
1A. What does it feel like under your hand or in your whole body? Is there pulsing, rocking, or temperature change? Stay for about a minute until there is a sign to move—a breath? A shudder? Or an emotion?
2. Place your hand on your forehead. Touch your neocortex where thinking, figuring, and analyzing take place. Do 1A.
3. Place your hand on your heart. Touch your heart where feelings and compassion live. Do 1A.
4. Place your hand on your belly. Touch your belly where your gut feelings live. They are often the first to dysregulate in trauma (sick to my stomach). Do 1A.

As you were tracking—brain, heart, and belly—what was prominent? What was closed down? What spoke to you? What helped you settle? As you practice this, you can become aware of more, different messages coming through.

With this tracking EX, you are seeking differences. Why? Because the trauma imprint is always the same: the same flashbacks, the same body patterns. Regular, everyday memories change, like the famous story of catching a fish. Each time you tell the story, the fish gets bigger. But trauma stays the same. It seems to last forever, which is also the view of a young child. Your body is the medium to inform you of your trauma. This tracking EX helps you see that change is possible. This is a valuable lesson, even if traumatic patterns are not overwhelming you in the moment.

Advanced tracking can be defined as follows:

> The capacity to sense oneself must become so refined that the individual can discriminate between physical sensation and the sensation of essential substance. It is not enough that the mind be quiet. It is also necessary for the body to be sensitive. The mind can be quiet while the body is deadened. The body has to be awakened…[2]

III – BODY MAP

EX – BODY MAP

Sensory awareness, cognition, and motor skills are all involved in the physicality of embodiment. Structure, function, and size are important when bringing attention to your body. It is often said in the trauma-resolution work, "Bring your attention to your body." But if that is colored by your idea of structure, function, and size, this idea is not clear yet. What you think the body looks like (or your "map") may not be an accurate picture of what is actually there. Details and dimensions may be off.

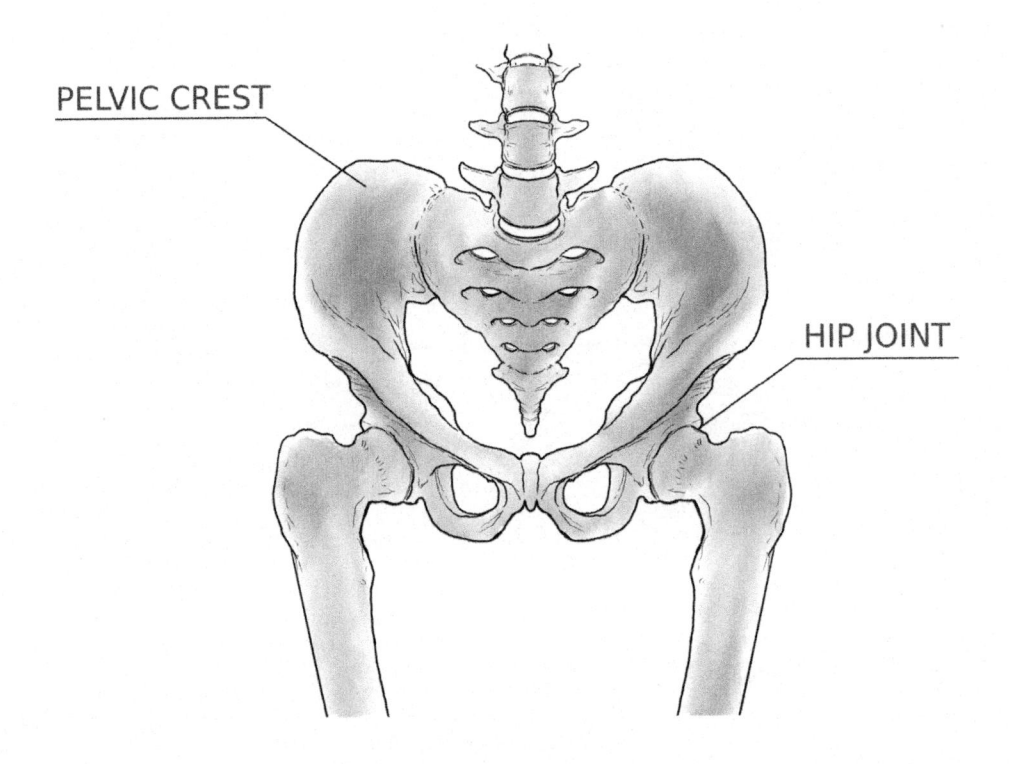

Pelvic Crest and Hip Joint

Where your hip joints are is often mapped incorrectly. It is not the pelvic crest.

Some people talk about diaphragmatic breathing and point to their belly. The diaphragm is up under the ribs and never drops below the ribs.

With developmental or shock trauma, the accuracy of one's body map may be off, creating a disconnect between thought, sensation, and movement. With correct guidance this map can be updated to create flowing, coordinated, and easeful movement. There is no need to study classical anatomy, but a few ideas of functional anatomy (that are presented in the EXploracises below, from head to toe) can be helpful.

EX – Head on the Pillow

For years I've noticed that sometimes I lie down to sleep or even just to rest, and while my head is on the pillow, it is nowhere near on the pillow. (I explain what I mean below.) I have also noticed a kind of tightness in my neck and many necks of people that I work with, observe, see, encounter, or talk to. I used to think that this tightness was an element of the startle response. As Frank Pierce Jones discovered with multi-strobe photography, the first element of the startle reflex response is to shorten the back neck muscles and pull your head back and down to your neck.[3] This is a main element of the teachings of the Alexander Technique.

One day, I decided to investigate my own neck tightness that I had observed for many years and had tried, unsuccessfully, to change. As I lay down, I realized that my head was nowhere near the pillow—my head was not supported. One of the basic HUMANUAL EXs is to receive support from the ground, given that you are on the planet.[4] With the tightness in my head on the pillow, I realized that I was holding my head up and not letting it rest on the pillow. I decided to ask for support and to imagine someone holding my head so I didn't have to. I imagined hands that I could trust to hold my head. I needed educated, open, connected, fleshy, supportive hands. They held my head so I didn't have to.

After a while, I realized that I was holding my head up off the planet to not fully arrive here, just the same as I had done with my feet on the ground receiving support. It was not the startle pattern. It was a failure to allow myself to be here fully on the planet. When I realized this, the connections between my head and my body, especially my shoulders, changed dramatically. I felt my whole body as one, as I had never felt before. In that moment of the oneness, I seemed to take off and float or fly through space and time. Solid but not solid. A very enjoyable experience almost like a balloon flying through space as the air slowly comes out. The correlation between my feet on the ground receiving support and my head on the ground receiving support was felt in a very new and deep way, leading my head to be on the pillow. Explore this for yourself.

EX – Jaw Movement

I had a wonderful singing teacher at the Lichtenberger Institute in Germany named Gisela Rohmert. I used to watch her move her mouth when she was watching a student sing; it was like she was chewing something, releasing her jaw with the movement. Try moving your mouth like you are chewing, with just your bottom jaw moving or do it with your head and jaw moving. It stimulates the fascial system in the whole body.

EX – Jaw Movement Clarified

1. Your jaw does not move efficiently when you use the large muscles on the sides of your neck. Jaw movement happens in two very tiny joints that are under your skull in front of your ear. The condyles of your jaw bone glide forward, like a drawer opening. Your jaw moves freely and lightly from there.
2. When you move your jaw this way, you can contact the relationship between your jaw and your pelvis.

III – BODY MAP

3. As you sit, lean your torso over your legs and let your head hang. Sometimes it is easier to feel your jaw release when your head is hanging upside down. In this position, it is also easier to connect your jaw and pelvis. Sit up and feel the results.
4. If you feel your jaw is tight, take a big bite from a sour apple. The movement and the saliva can help to release your jaw.
5. A tight jaw is often associated with anger, wanting to say something but holding it in. As you exhale, open your mouth and let out a deep sigh, or even growl sounds to dissipate the anger. The deep sigh can release down through your whole torso to your pelvis.
6. Note that a necktie tightens your neck and jaw, as it separates **head and body.**

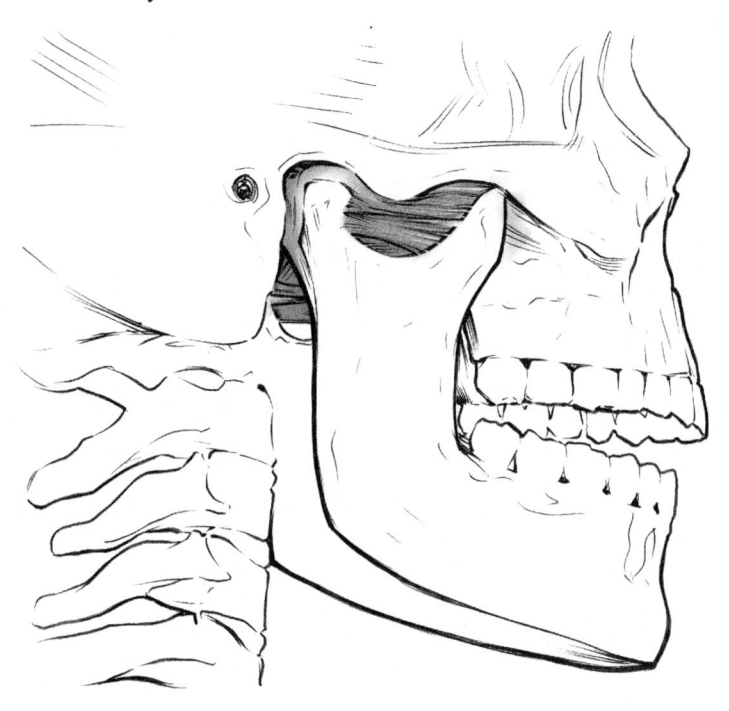

Jaw

EXPLORACISES

EX – Tongue

There are many opinions about where the tongue wants to rest. Some say it rests on the floor of the mouth, and some say it rests on the roof. From my many years of exploration, I have come to the conclusion that for the best results for inner health and upright posture, your tongue rests on the roof of your mouth. When the tongue rests on the floor of your mouth, it creates a downward pressure on your whole system and often juts the head forward.

Fascial continuity runs from the tongue and jaw muscles down through the whole body to the inner arch of the foot, engaging a core support. Paying attention to your tongue posture, by sealing your tongue to the roof of your mouth, creates a fascial rudder to the toes. Be sure to include the back of your tongue connecting to the soft palate.

Practice oral posture with oral pharyngeal exercises:

1. Put the back of your tongue to the roof of your mouth.
2. Push your tongue to the roof of your mouth while swallowing. Don't push teeth.
3. *Mewing* is a face-reconstructing technique that aims to change your jawline's shape. The process involves keeping your tongue on the roof of your mouth. Mewing used to be exclusively for mouth, jaw, and dental issues, but now, my seven-year-old grandson tells me, it is a TikTok sensation for looking cool.
4. Shut your mouth with your teeth almost touching. Tongue on the roof of your mouth. Lightly touch your teeth with your tongue up.

EX – Shoulder Float

1. Let your right shoulder float.
2. Let it float forward, backward, down, and up.
3. Repeat 1 and 2 with your left shoulder.
4. Explore letting them float together. One forward, one back, or any combination you like.

EX – Pelvis and Sitting Bones

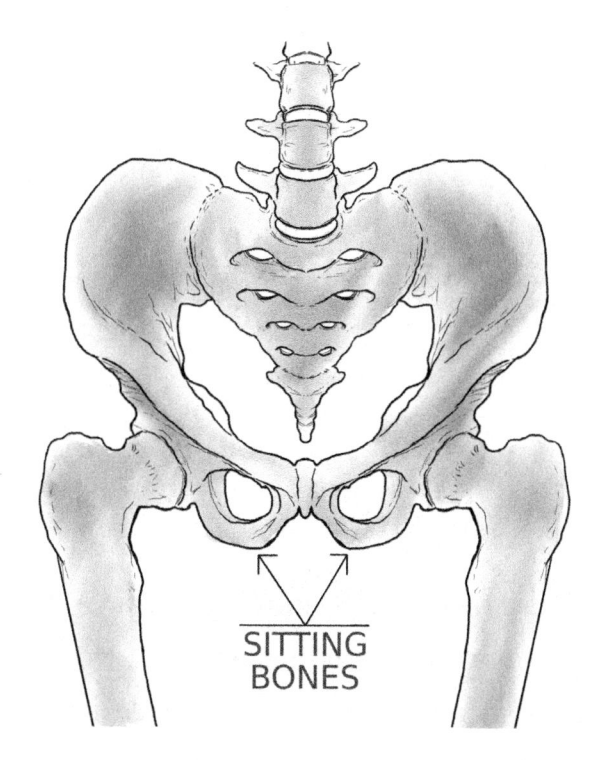

Sitting Bones

1. The bones at the bottom of your pelvis are called the sitting bones. They are like little rockers with a V-shaped bottom. Many people sit on their legs and not on their sit bones. When

you sit on your sit bones, your legs can be free. Sitting bones are like the feet of the torso.

2. When sitting, many tend to slump back as if defeated or put down. Others lean forward, over-arched, as in looking for recognition or approval. Explore both.

3. Rock back and forth and end up sitting on the center of your rockers. Can you find the balance where you are awake, upright, and alert? Are you comfortable there? Or scared or vulnerable (able to be wounded)?

4. Many people, mistakenly, rock back and forth from their waist instead of their hip sockets. The waist is not an anatomical reality. You will not find it in an anatomy book. It is a fashion concept. The anatomical reality is your spine, connected to your pelvis, that functions as one whole unit, and you pivot from your hip sockets to bend forward.

EX – Legs

1. The floor is the fixed object. Your legs are able to move at your ankles, knees, and hips.

2. Your legs move from the hip joints (just above the sitting bones). They do not move from the pelvic crest; that is much higher. Also, the thigh bone comes in from the side, not front to back, as many people think.

3. The knee is a space between upper and lower leg bones, and it bends in one direction only.

4. There is mobility at the ankle joint, where the foot bones meet the lower leg bones.

5. When there is a lot of pressure downward to compress the legs, the nerves have reduced sensation. When we ask someone, "What sensation do you feel?" and they say, "None," it is accurate as there is so much collapse.

EX – Sole to Soul

1. The sole of the foot meets the Earth. The reflexes at the bottom of your feet send messages to the rest of your body to adjust to the shifting terrain. So when you step on an uneven surface, your body adjusts.
2. The soul of the being meets the Earth and Heaven. The reflexes then connect to the light-filled energetic body we all have.

After this somatic journey, with your body map, let's see where you land. As you are reading, do you feel any constriction in your jaw, neck, shoulders, ribs, pelvic area, knees, or feet? If you say "no" to all of these, write to me. I will send you a free book. Modern life has so much stress that we all constrict, and this limits our breathing and functioning. Correcting your body map can reduce the constrictions.

IV – SOMATIC PRINCIPLES

EX – SOMATICS of the Living Body

We are somatic creatures. We feel each other and ourselves. Touch is always mutual. As babies, we feel our way through the environment to understand our world. This process of scanning or awareness is always on, checking the surroundings for safety, danger, or ways to get our needs met. When we are upset or need help as babies or children, our nervous system gets jangled, and our caregiver is supposed to give us help or co-regulation (an interactive process providing support). With that, the nervous system can relax and feel nourished or satisfied. If we do not get help, we stop feeling, as the feelings are too painful to manage.

- Find a small connection that feels safe. Maybe a friend or your dog? Notice and encourage the physical sensations that arise.
- Books are filled with advice on what we "should" do to feel better. Instead, do an activity that soothes your unique and unfolding system (take a bath, go for a walk, etc.).

- If you realize there has been a rupture in a relationship, do what feels right to repair any breach in connection.
- When you are observing yourself, do so with compassion, and not with a cold judging lens. If you observe coldly, you leave out feelings, and then you are doing what the untended baby needed to do, which was to not feel.

EX – Objectifying the Body

When we look closely, we see that we tend to objectify our bodies. We often say "my body did this or that," "it" tightened or got an illness. It is not like that. Your body is not a static object that you feel. You don't feel your body... what you feel or become aware of is your current state of organization—how you are organizing yourself, including body, cognition, and emotion.

What are you organized to do? That is the question. See what happens when you try these states—do any fit your mode of organization?

1. What do you look like when you are rushing (being late)?
2. Worrying?
3. Repressing anger?
4. Reset. Return to center.
5. How are you organized when you are enjoying (friends, your favorite hobby)?
6. Discovering (like in a retreat or reading a good book)?
7. Being curious, listening to observe what you are doing?
8. There is bidirectional communication between mind and body, one system of wholeness. Every thought is like a bath or wave of

energy to your tissues. Thoughts are biologically active. Thus the phrase "the issue is in the tissue."

EX – Are You Thinking, Feeling, Sensing, or Doing?

1. Think. (cognitive)
2. Feel. (general tone)
3. Sense. (specifically defined)
4. Do. (more active)
5. Can you tell the difference between 1, 2, 3, and 4? They each provide a different physical experience. Thinking tends to ignore the body. Feeling provides a general tonus. Sensing is a very specific, often localized, inner movement. Doing is a more active physical activity.

> "When you think you're thinking, you're feeling; when you think you're feeling, you're doing."
>
> —F.M. Alexander

EX – Orienting with Movement

Orienting brings us to the *now* moment, looking around and wondering, *Is it safe or safe enough? Is there connection here? Can I feel at home? Do I belong?* When people have experienced trauma, or a series of overwhelming emotions, they respond to their environment in one of two ways: they are either hypervigilant, looking around all the time, typically nervously, and the sternocleidomastoid (SCM) muscle is overactive; or they are the opposite of this, not wanting to

IV – SOMATIC PRINCIPLES

investigate their surroundings or engage with others because of the potential for danger—in which case the sternocleidomastoid is often stuck, limiting head movement. Practicing orienting can help both. Orient for safety and/or connection. We are visually orienting in this EXploracise, one of many ways an organism can orient. Before you begin, touch the large muscle (SCM) that runs down the side of your neck, as you turn your head.

1. Sit. Turn your head to the right, then left. Feel your neck muscles moving. Which side is more comfortable? See objects in your space. As you look around, you may find that habitual vigilance makes you feel safe or unsafe.
2. Turn your head and let your shoulders move. Return back to center. Do it on the other side.
3. Turn so much that your hips rotate, and your low back moves, to see behind you. Do it on the other side.
4. Stand. Turn your head, looking, and let your shoulders move—your arms can move to stretch, welcome, or fight. What happens to you? Do your arms want to hug and reach with longing or punch with rage? Do the other side.
5. Return to center. Then turn so much that your hips rotate. The muscles in your hips will activate your legs to just walk—for a stroll, stomp, a run to get you out and away—or could possibly freeze, if you think danger is approaching.
6. Then settle. Recognize what is now in the room that you never saw before. Notice that you might be a little less held at your joints, muscles, and fascia. Stories imprinted on your fascia can change too.

EX – Early Orienting

I notice that many people look down a lot, and they rarely inhabit the space above their head, thus never fully inhabiting uprightness.

1. How comfortable are you living in or expanding into the space above your head?
2. Are you able to be comfortable with the space over your head? And expanding into your full stature?
3. Can you look up and free yourself into the space above?
4. Or is it scary and you want to pull your head down and narrow your visual field? Narrowing the field of attention is often a prelude to looking for danger.

When babies look around, they are looking freely for a breast, with neck rotating easily, and the space overhead is available. But for many, a breast or bottle was shoved into their mouth when it was convenient for the mother/caregiver or when the doctor told them to. The rooting reflex, with a free neck, looking for the breast, does not want to be limited. I wonder how much of this early pull down influences our comfort and desire to be upright later in life.

IV – SOMATIC PRINCIPLES

EX – Standing Patterns

1. Where do you stand habitually—on what part of your foot—balls, sides, or heels?
2. Explore…the forward pattern leaning on your toes that is often present when…*I want something or I want to be heard or I need to go somewhere.* Return to center.
3. Explore…the backward pattern leaning on your heels. This is often present when…*I want to be a little behind everything, no thank you, hiding, organized to retreat a little.* Return to center.
4. Explore…with your feet to find center. Find equal pressure with the balls of your foot and your heels. This affects breath, mood, outlook, and rhythm. It is not one solid place. There is always some movement on this planet, a slight rocking or figure 8. You have a center. The center in you connects to the center of others and the universe. Where is what you would call your center?

EX – Dynamic Opposition

The concept of oppositions in relation to the body and movement is a very important one. It is not possible for everything to go in one direction. There are oppositions within the body and with the body and an outside object, like the floor. The idea is visible in movement, if we go back to 18th-century Vienna and watch the swirling partners waltzing. The partners oppose each other by leaning back, but then move as one flowing unit. The dynamic opposition creates unity.

1. Feel your body being dropped down to the Earth, and at the same time reach up to the Heavens.
2. Hold your arms out to the side parallel to the floor and feel the stretch between your hands, pulling in opposite directions. If you don't tighten your arms, can you feel the lightness?
3. As you breathe out, your sternum and spine aim up, while your ribs drape down, fueling your breath.
4. If you can find a partner, try the waltzing!

EX – Boundary

Many people understand the need for mental boundaries, such as saying no to a request or saying no for the purpose of self-care. Let's explore the physicality of boundaries. Because, as physician Gabor Maté states in his seminal book *When the Body Says No*, if we don't say "NO," our body will.

1. Stand. Explore your kinesphere, the space you can reach around you as you stand.
2. Explore with your hands what the space around you feels like. What is it like to reach above your head, behind you, all around you? Touch it or imagine it.
3. Where is your comfortable boundary—is it with your hands close to your body, or with your hands extended as far as they can reach?
4. Explore creating a boundary with your hands motioning to stop as you say "NO." Your hands are pushing away.

IV – SOMATIC PRINCIPLES

5. From a balanced support, for any kind of violation, as your hands push away, you can say, "This is my space. Nobody and nothing comes in unless I say so. No bully, or critical thoughts, insults, or microaggressions, NO!!" No is not just a no—it makes room for a yes somewhere else. Find your "YES." Boundaries want to be permeable and porous, not rigid. If we have healthy boundaries, we are not overwhelmed.

V – NUANCES OF PHYSICALITY

Stretch has become the S word. In many circles of movement or education, stretching as we know it has been called ineffective and dangerous. So why do it at all? The question comes up: Do I need to stretch every day or at all?

Muscles have two functions: they contract and they stop contracting. They do not actually stretch, but they release into length. When you stretch a muscle, the first thing that happens is the nervous system says, "Yikes, what is happening? You are coming apart," and the muscle contracts. This is called the stretch reflex. If you engage the stretch reflex, you will never lengthen a muscle.

Muscles themselves do not DO anything. I—which includes my fascial system, nervous system, circulatory system, musculoskeletal system, respiratory system, etc.—will be living in a state of ease or a state of effort, and my muscles and connective tissue will reflect either state. When I detect danger, these systems want to protect me, so I contract muscles. That said, I do not DO anything. I become one unit of contracted muscles: mind, body, emotion, and vibration as one frequency pulsing together. Like the firefly story.

If you want to "stretch," you consciously decide to release a muscle into its full length. You and all your systems agree this is okay when you realize that you are not under threat. When you are under threat, real or perceived, your muscles will contract to protect and over-effort, in a sympathetic state of defense.

EX – Stretch Muscles or Release Connective Tissues

1. Stretch any muscle. See what you sense. Stop.
2. Recognize that you are not in danger by orienting, then release that same muscle and surrounding connective tissue into length. Stop.
3. Note the difference between 1 and 2.
4. Reread "Pandiculation" in Chapter 1.

EX – Pain and Rhythm

1. Choose a physical pain and bring your attention to the pain.
2. Find the tensing or constriction under the pain.
3. Move into the constriction a tiny bit with gentle pulsing, not tightening.
4. The constriction will most likely open a bit to expansion with a breath or sigh.
5. Go back and forth between the contraction and the expansion a few times.

6. Feel the flow and rhythm between them, so there is less polarity between them. You want the rhythm to be the dominant player, not the pain.
7. You can stay at the edge of the expansion and explore small micro-movements to move into it. It may have an image of a wall or barrier of some sort. Let the small micro-movements shift the barrier. Very gently. No forcing, shoving, or MANipulating. Stay aware that the barrier has a relationship to the original constriction and the rhythm.
8. You are a living matrix, always vibrating in rhythmic pulsation.

EX – Default Mode Network (DMN),
based on the work of Dr. Ruth Lanius

Experiences and self-related thoughts are represented neurobiologically by a large-scale cortical network located along the brain's midline and referred to as the default mode network (DMN). The DMN is the part of the brain that is engaged when you are at rest. In a magnetic resonance imaging (MRI) brain scanner, if you have no history of major trauma, you can relax and not think of anything in particular. The DMN is activated and connected. It allows you to know what you want to do and where you want to go, and what your values are, or what music you want to hear. This can be beneficial, but if the DMN gets overactive, it can begin to ruminate excessively about past and future, causing worry and self-blame.

In daily life, the DMN activates the parts of your brain called the posterior cingulate (PCC), medial prefrontal cortex, and parts of the parietal lobe. The DMN helps you to know what you are feeling and where you are in space. Right now, I am in my house or outside on a bicycle. Each will get a different sensation or feeling in your body. At rest, the DMN is active and connected in healthy individuals, and not active and connected in traumatized individuals.

After a traumatic experience, the core sense of self is disturbed. People who have traumatic stress have very few connections within the DMN when they are quiet. They don't have a strong sense of self, or feel very alive. They don't feel energized when they are just living. When you put some types of traumatized people in a situation of threat, the DMN comes "online," and they feel enlivened and more like themselves being in a state of threat than being in a state of quiet.[5]

EX – The Moment Before Sleep

1. Stay there. Don't sleep.
2. Feel the edge—between being consciously awake and leaving to go into another state of consciousness.
3. Become aware of your body. Perhaps a wavy, vague body image will be with you—of you watching, barely conscious. A conscious ending to your present state, instead of just becoming unaware.
4. Your eyelids slide gently down to close your eyes, slowly.
5. Feel the gel-like liquid that is between your eyes and eyelids.
6. Feel the roundness of your eyes. Feel the curve.
7. Feel what happens when your top eyelids meet the bottom.
8. How does that affect your whole body?
9. Then let your whole eyeball rest in the socket and fall to the back of your head.
10. Picture yourself in a deep dark cave for internal earthly peace, or sleeping under the stars to be wrapped in the heavenly skies.
11. Drift off to sleep.

EXPLORACISES

> "Ain't it just like the night to play tricks
> when you're trying to be so quiet."
>
> —*Bob Dylan*

Sleep researcher Thomas Wehr removed test participants from every possible form of artificial light from dusk to dawn, so they went to sleep in a natural environment. He discovered after one month that the hormone prolactin reached elevated levels in the participants. Prolactin creates a feeling of security, quietness, and peace. And it is intimately, and biologically, tied to the dark, so mammals are quietly at rest while they're sleeping.[6]

EX – Reaction Time

In a Western movie, when the hero and the villain face off in a gun battle, the villain draws first, but the hero is always able to beat him to the first shot and win. The hero's nervous system responds to the situation and organizes his muscles and fascia to operate without voluntary control. This is faster than the villain's deliberate and conscious voluntary action. The brilliance of the built-in system.

EX – Tremor

When you have a fast tremor or tic, after it finishes, move slowly and consciously in and out of the direction of the tremor. You are listening to what it wants to do, and you are adding a conscious element to it.

V – NUANCES OF PHYSICALITY

EX – Dynamic Stability

1. While you are standing, find something solid or stable to bring your awareness to—for example, a tree or a pyramid. You can put it inside or outside you.
2. Make a motion with your body to represent it. For the tree, with your hands show roots going down and branches going up. For a pyramid, sketch the shape from a point at the top, down to the ground or to your sides.
3. Let it get bigger and bigger. Roots down and branches up. Or point concentrated at the top and base wide at the bottom.
4. Stop the large outer movement, return to a neutral stable stance, and explore the movement you just did in small micro-movements. Go down a little. Back to neutral. Go up. Back to neutral. Etc.
5. This motion with awareness is a good way to stabilize and to experience your capacity for dynamic stability.

EX – Vibration and Frequency

Everything in the universe vibrates. The vibrations send out waves that can be measured. A wave that goes up, down, up equals one wavelength. The number of times a wave repeats per unit of time is called frequency, and this range is measured in hertz (Hz). One hertz means one cycle per second. Things vibrate or oscillate at different speeds. The amount of movement up, down, up in one second can be a variety of hertz.

EXPLORACISES

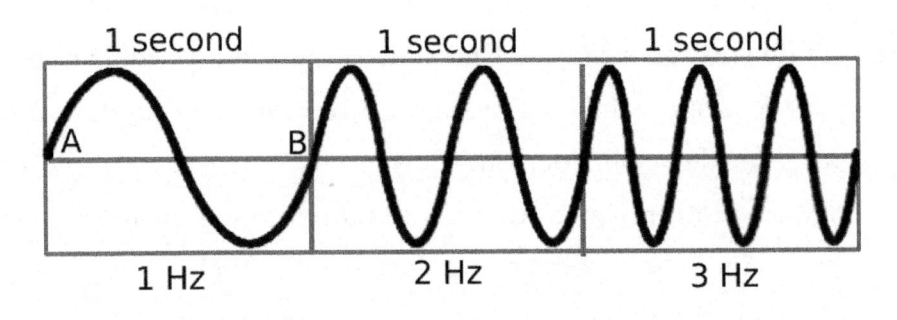

Hertz

1. When you are calm, and enjoying friends and good food, you vibrate one frequency.
2. When you are activated or in danger, your system begins to vibrate at another frequency.

- According to existing research, the natural frequency of a human standing body is about 7.5–8 Hz, also known as the Schumann resonance, the frequency of the Earth, the documented fundamental electromagnetic "heartbeat" of Earth. Research says that music tuned to the frequency of 432 Hz, a multiple or octave of 8 Hz, is easier to listen to, brighter, clearer, and contains more inherent dynamic range. And in some cases, it lowers blood pressure and heart rate of listeners.[7]
- Dr. Stephen Porges has created music to calm your nervous system and promote overall wellbeing. Discover the power of polyvagal music and experience the soothing effects with Safe and Sound Protocol and Sonocea, the Sound of Science, created together with Anthony Gorry.[8]

V – NUANCES OF PHYSICALITY

- The human ear can hear between 20 and 20,000 Hz (20 kHz), but it is most sensitive to everything that happens between 250 and 5,000 Hz.
- The fundamental frequency is the primary pitch of our voices. The typical human voice frequency range is between 85 and 255 Hz, with adult males generally having a lower range (around 85–155 Hz) and adult females having a higher range (around 165–255 Hz). The voice also produces higher frequencies called harmonics, which add richness and character to the sound.
- Middle C is around 256 Hz (also a multiple of 8).
- Humans hum around 128 Hz, which is C below middle C, a harmonic. Try it in the next EX.

EX – HUMM 1

We all have an inner frequency, a vibration that keeps us alive. It is the vibration of our tune or unique song.

1. Start to hum. Become aware of the inner vibration it produces.
2. Put your fingers on your throat. Feel your vocal cords slightly vibrating, awakening your sensory world.
3. Check other places in your body. Feel your vibration. Each body part is different. How does it vibrate in your head? Where in your head? Where is there less vibration?
4. Cup your hands at your mouth as you hum. How does it affect you?
5. Hum one verse of a song you like.
6. The HUMM releases nitric oxide and dilates blood vessels.

7. The vagus nerve passes through the vocal cords and the middle ear. The vibrations of humming influence your nervous system states.
8. Bees make a humming sound, and they beat their wings to the key of C. This frequency resonates at 256 Hz, which can produce harmonizing effects on the human mind and reset the brain out of cognitive dissonance. Biophysics, or physics applied to biological systems, is part of a new medical model, proving that nature can facilitate healing.

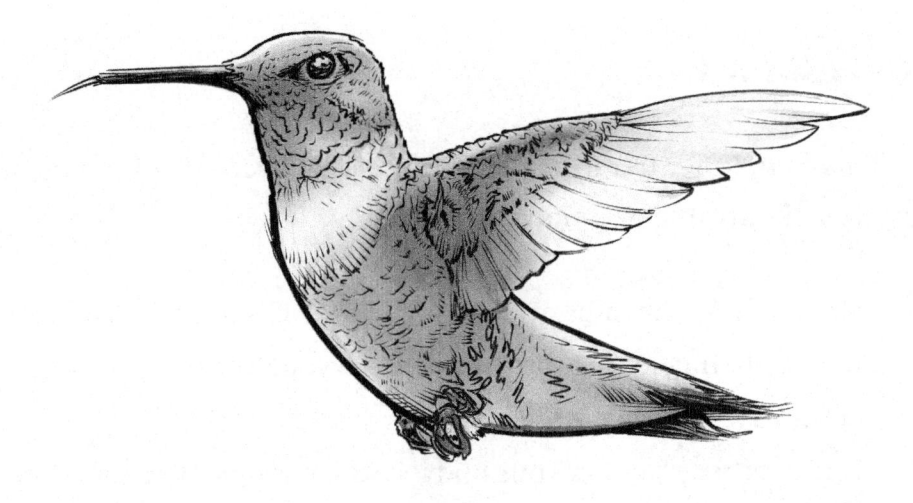

Hummingbird

EX – HUMM 2

When humming:

1. In front…start with your hand or hands on your neck.
2. Move your hands down little by little as the vibration spreads to your chest. This vibrates the vagus nerve that goes from head to belly. End with your hand(s) on your belly.
3. In back…start at the back of your head and feel the vibration.
4. Move the hands down as you are able, and end with your hands on your mid-back at the kidney area, near your adrenal glands.

Nikola Tesla said,

> "If you want to find the secrets of the universe, think in terms of energy, frequency, and vibration."

VI – SUSPENSION

My Dream: Imagine or Picture This for Yourself

Somebody was holding me up. Up, so my feet were off the ground about two inches. I was hanging by my ears. It was not uncomfortable. As I stayed there, different parts of me let go. When my pelvis let go, the person holding me acknowledged it with a "that's it." And there was this immediate connection between my head and my body. My body was suspended from my head, but just enough let go to have my head and body connected in the most unifying way.

It was like when you hold a cat by the nape of its neck. Holding by the back of the neck lets the head release slightly forward. And bingo, the body is suspended from the head. The body can let go and connect more. Interesting that is how animals hold their young ones.

I don't really like to write about "head" and "body," but in this case it does make things quite clear. The detached middle ear bones seem to play a part here because you are holding near that area. The connection seems to come from that space of the detached ear bones, allowing the connection between what is above and below it. The slight expansion

VI – SUSPENSION

invites head and body to become one continuous tensegrity structure, an inner soft white flexible cloud. Like my dream.

EX – Suspension

Part of healthy, human, wellbeing wholeness is a kind of elasticity or suspension. I spoke of the elastic suit we all wear, the layer of fascia or connective tissue just under the skin. But as research and anecdote show, trauma often creates a scar or a rigid protective barrier, a constriction that prevents elasticity.

There are two types of (mechanical) voluminous structural systems, a compression system and a suspension system. A compression system is bricks stacked up, compressed on each other. Our human skeleton does not stack up, as there are no flat surfaces to rest on. A suspension system is an expanded system—everything is slightly expanded, with forces pushing in and forces pushing out in a dynamic balance, as we saw in the tensegrity section (Chapter 1). Recent research tells us that our inner biology is a suspension system right down to our cells. Constriction interferes with suspension.

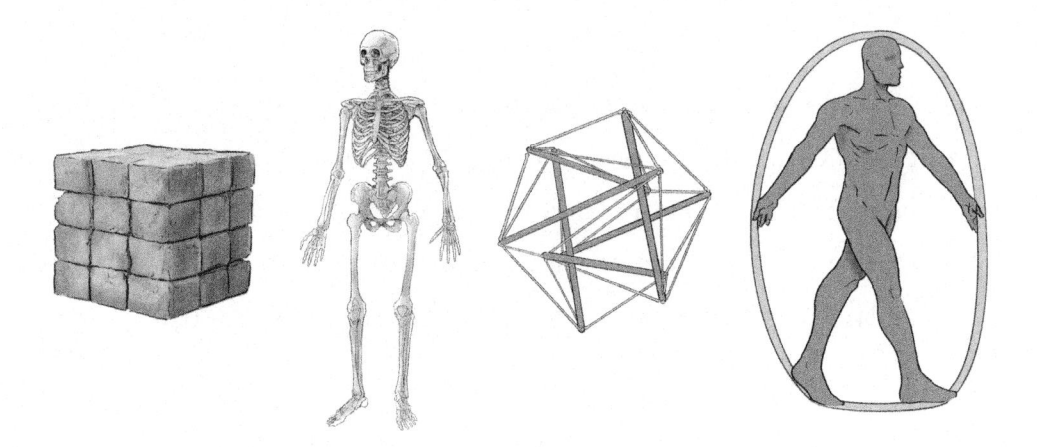

Bricks stack, skeletons do not.
Tensegrity is tensile, humans are also.

EXPLORACISES

1. What do you notice as you sit? Usually there are some places of comfort, and some of discomfort. Find one place of constriction, not the worst. Constriction is the first response to a shocking event in the body…sticking together, the body's attempt to hold it all together or protect.
2. Picture yourself as a woven web of three-dimensional fabric that is pinched or gathered where the constriction is.
3. Is it collapsed, or pulled with fear or repressed anger?
4. DON'T fix it. But experience it. Be curious. The implicit memory says it has to be this way. So, we have compassion. I so get you needed this.
5. Peek at it from a distance. Get to know it.
6. How big? Shape? Color?
7. Is there any movement? You can't stop contraction. You can't fight against contraction. But maybe it can be changed.
8. Move into it.
9. Is it affected by breath?
10. Go back and forth between breath and contraction.
11. Perhaps it shifts on its own toward suspension or elasticity or wholeness. Or maybe now there is space around it.
12. How do you feel when you have a bit more space inside? Is it okay? Go back and forth. Touch in and come out. Perhaps the lack of suspension or elasticity that constrictions leave you with can be changed. Yes, there is pain and suffering, and yes, your elasticity is there waiting for you to join your wholeness.

VII – SUPPORT

All infants need to be held by a caregiver. Picture a mother figure holding a baby in their arms. If the caregiver is texting or cooking or doing some other activity, they may not be giving the child enough support, attention, or holding. When a child feels not held, they take it upon themselves and interpret the situation to mean *"I need to hold myself up,"* thereby creating some kind of stiffening, or held pattern. Later in life, this constrictive pattern may lead to thinking and believing *"I need to do it all myself."*

There are many kinds of somatic support—a friend may put a hand on your back, a colleague might give you a supportive look or thumbs-up, or a stranger may help you with an act of kindness. I am acknowledging another kind of support, the support from the universe. There are forces and energies that we are not consciously aware of, fields of energy—a built-in support that is already there. We can bring awareness to this internal universal support that moves within and around us.

EX – Support

As life on Planet Earth has it, we live in a gravitational field, and we need to adapt to that. Most people do not think about that at all, but it does matter. You don't worry about it all the time, but there is a part of you that is taking care of that for you. You don't want to fall over. There is a big sky above and a big Earth below. We are connected to both.

There is gravity and antigravity. Gravity has a bad name. People think that slumping and bad posture are because of gravity. But it is not gravity. Look at healthy children. They don't sit like that. If gravity did it, everybody would be slumped over. Gravity comes down with a force toward the Earth, and the Earth is spinning and giving off a centrifugal force upward. Plants and trees grow with an upward force toward the sun. The body has a set of muscles taking it away from gravity, the extensors, and toward gravity, the flexors.

We love verticality. Who told children to stand up? As you read in Chapter 1, in physics the upward force is called the ground reaction force, GRF. The amount of weight you put into the Earth is matched by an upward force. Gravity and antigravity meet. It is a vital interface because it is how we meet the planet, to live our life and have our human experiences.

Trauma or overwhelm knocks us off this support. When we are living with the effects of a traumatic incident, we lose our support, both literally and figuratively. Our equilibrium, balance, and rhythm are often disturbed. When a traumatic incident happened, maybe no one was there to take care of, to protect, or to support us. The organized biological coherence was gone. Support is a key element on many levels. The word is made up of *sub*, 'from below,' plus *portare*, 'carry.' Support is to carry from below. Let's practice and find support.

VII – SUPPORT

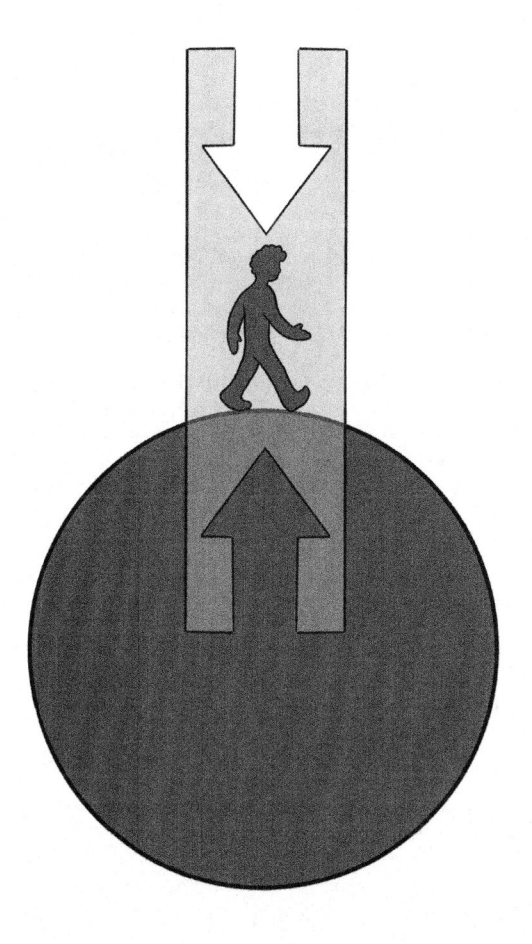

Support from below

For our journey with support, recognize the layer just under your skin made of fascia that we have explored—the continuous three-dimensional matrix of structural support, the elastic envelope. This multidirectional, multidimensional fascial arrangement both supports and allows you to move in multiple directions.

EXPLORACISES

EX – Stand with Support

This EXploracise is not about gross motor movements. Allow yourself to respond with small changes. Support from the ground connects to your inner support.

1. Bring your awareness to the bottoms of your feet.
2. Let the bottoms of your feet feel the floor (or the ground if you are outside). Notice how and where they meet the floor. Some parts have contact with the floor, and others are often pulling up off the floor. Just notice; don't try to fix anything.
3. Now become aware that the ground is under you, and allow the floor to support you. Notice how the rest of your body responds to the support.
4. Let the support come up through your body.
5. Let your ankles be free enough to receive that support from the ground.
6. Let your knees be free enough to let the support come through.
7. Let your hip sockets be less held, so that the support can come up through them.
8. Continue to your lower, middle, and upper torso, and your whole back.
9. Spread out your arms, so your arms are supported by the ground.
10. Let your neck and head be free, floating upward from the ground.
11. Let your eyes look where they want, as you see shapes and colors.

VII – SUPPORT

If you don't understand that you are supported, you will try to hold yourself up, often with your shoulders. But if you understand that you are a whole being, and on the ground—meaning that you will not fall down because you are already supported by the ground—then there is no need to hold yourself up.

This is not the same as what most people call "grounding," which often has a strong *down* component. My teaching is about meeting the ground, not to go down and only "root" oneself but to open and receive an upward force. Heaven and Earth meeting in synchronized embodiment.

I taught this support EX in a group class at a conference. After the practice, when I asked for comments, a woman raised her hand. She said she was surprised that she actually felt support. I nodded, as I was not surprised. She went on to say, "No, you don't understand—I have Ehlers-Danlos syndrome [hypermobile joints], and so normally every time I stand, I need to put out a tremendous amount of effort and energy, just to stand and not fall down. And in this moment, I did not need all that work to stand. The support held me up." She was grateful for the new experience.

EX – Quick Support

1. Contact what is under you.
2. Recognize and receive support.
3. Allow breath.
4. Look around to connect to the environment.
5. Do this with bare feet on the ground, to meet the life-giving energy of the Earth more directly.

EX – Gradation of Support

I was at the beach with my two-year-old grandson, and we were standing at the edge of the ocean as the waves were breaking. The waves were big, and he needed support to not get knocked over. I held him and caught him when he needed it. Little by little, as he needed less support, I loosened my contact.

1. Picture yourself in this situation.
2. What would it be like to have someone tuned to your every need and supporting you?
3. And for them to leave you free when you do not need support?

EX – Fall into the Environment

1. Picture yourself falling onto a raft on the water. Of course, the raft and water become support for you.
2. Now actually stand up. As you stand, let your feet fall to the ground and recognize that the ground becomes support.
3. As you stand, let yourself fall *upward*—go up and out into the environment. The environment now supports you. A new support, falling upward.
4. Stay connected to the ground as you fall up, and watch the small changes. This might give you a taste of your Egypt body (Chapter 2, section III).

VII – SUPPORT

EX – Bracing Pattern and Support

Your bracing pattern is unique to you. It includes every thought, feeling, emotion, and interaction that you ever had and maybe even more, including those of your ancestors. These patterns often start when people are young with needs being met or not, such as the need to be held and nurtured. If nobody did it, the system has to compensate. It shows up later in life when something difficult happens. When we need to protect ourselves from something "outside," we brace. The bracing prevents all kinds of stimuli from entering, not just the negative or overwhelming.

We try to let go of the bracing, but somehow it does not work. It will not let go, because it is part of a bigger picture. It will not let go because it needs to be replaced by something before it can change. This is where support comes in and is crucial—support from a person or situation or support from the group, the planet, the Earth that we are part of. Allow the ground to support you, a tiny bit at a time. And the bracing can then release a bit. The support is there first. Then the bracing can shift a little, instead of bracing for the next disaster. You cannot be holding on to bracing and letting go to support at the same time.

1. What does the bracing pattern look like in your neck? Your arms? Legs? Torso?
2. Stay with your bracing pattern for at least a few minutes every day. Don't try to change it. But be with it. Listen to the story it tells. Acknowledge it. Talk to it. Not at it. As you talk to yourself and look at what you are doing, the subconscious self comes to consciousness with the invitation. We then see that we have subconscious movement, conscious aware movement,

and emotionally touched movement, all related to the bracing pattern, and wanting to receive support.

EX – Doing - Non-Doing

Another way to understand the bracing pattern is to see it in terms of effort and no effort, or doing and non-doing. Many of us live our lives "doing" most of the time, getting things done. We rarely explore what non-doing has to offer. But our system can manifest both of these contrasting pathways. Both exist in our daily experience. Although not exactly the same, we can see the similarity with doing-being, voluntary-involuntary, conscious-subconscious—all the pairs contain an element of effort and an element of no effort.

1. Breath is probably the most obvious. Watch yourself breathe voluntarily or consciously.
2. Stop.
3. Allow your breath to happen involuntarily or subconsciously. I call it a *being breath*. Very different.

Go back and forth a few times. Switching from one to the other allows a deeper connection to the energetic and subtle body. More possibilities.

Try it with your hands.

1. Become aware of the tightening in your hands, always actively holding on to something.
2. Stop.
3. Let your hands settle into their resting position. Slightly cupped or arched. Very different from the doing, holding mode.

VII – SUPPORT

Try it with your eyes.

1. Eyes so often strain to see. They work in doing mode even when they are closed.
2. Stop.
3. Let your eyes just be. Not looking for someone or something. Let them fall into non-doing mode.

There is so much experience and information available to us from our subconscious, non-doing, involuntary self. With this EXploracise, you may need to go slowly, as deeper trauma patterns may emerge, because we are doing or holding for a reason.

EX – Aware of Wear and Tear

Years ago, I had neighbors from hell, the most selfish, inconsiderate people I had ever met. One day, they sent me a nasty email. When I read the email, I realized that they had totally ignored all my requests, and the information I provided, and assumed that they would just carry on in their nasty selfish way.

I felt my insides lift off from myself and shake and tremble. I lost my appetite, got confused, lost, angry and furious, and helpless all at the same time. I noticed that this energy pulled me up off my legs around my midcalf region. I was totally disconnected from my lower legs. The upper three-quarters were in a tizzy. I was separated from my support, from my essence, separated from my connected self and my innate organization, my expanded self.

In that moment, I realized how dangerous this is for my wellbeing—to be so physically disconnected from my Self. I was in global high activation. My whole system was supercharged away from itself. I saw it. I felt it. How would I get back?

It felt like we have a certain amount of "wellbeing capital," and that you should not spend or touch that. But in this moment, I was spending it. Not good. My nervous-system capital was draining out. For me, when in doubt…meditate. For others, maybe contemplate, or sit quietly with yourself, or walk or run and be active.

As I meditated, I saw and felt the pull so clearly. Definitely pulled off my support. It seemed to make sense to go to my support. That immediately reminded my system of my innate connection to myself and the universe. Little by little, I was able to stay with that and heal the place where I ripped apart from myself.

I also explored some details of my nervous system. I let my arms fight a little, to defend myself from this onslaught of lies from them. I pushed them and their ideas away. I also used my legs to walk and run away from the building. These movements connected me more to myself, and my innate wellbeing. The activity took me out of helplessness and into the sympathetic nervous system, and agency. Always returning to my support. My wholeness was there, eventually, taking me into ventral vagal. Now I could see the sun shine.

CHAPTER 4

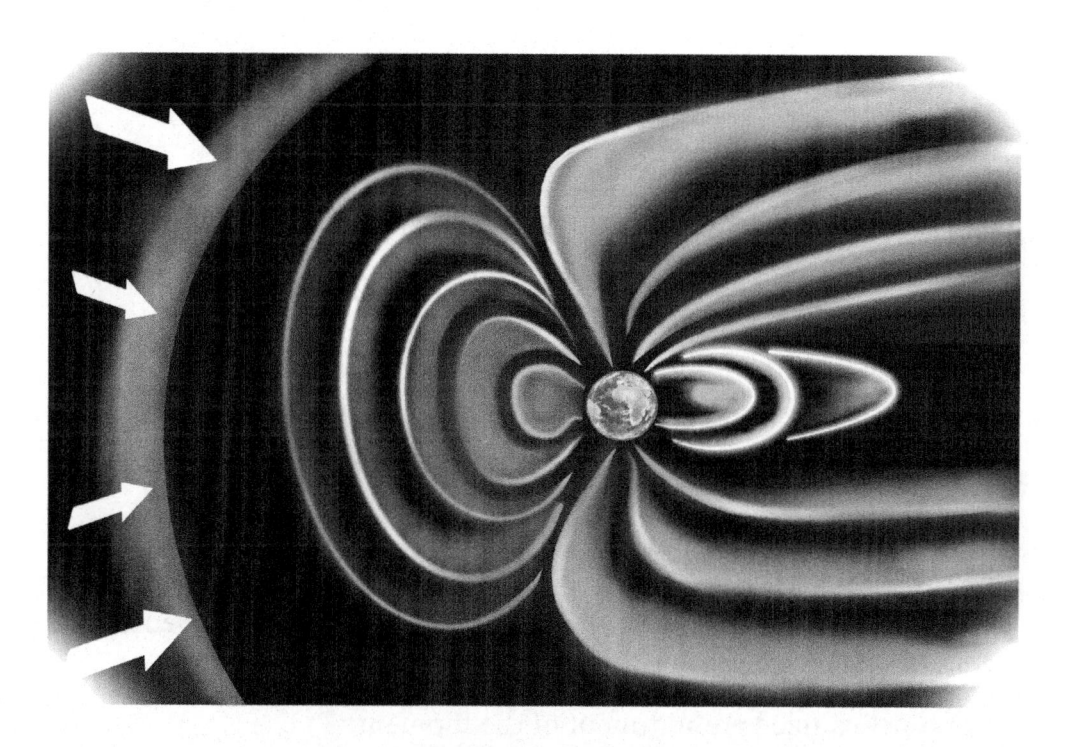

TAKING EXPLORACISES
TO THE NEXT LEVEL

I – DEEPER DIVE EXPLORACISES

Get ready to dive into the depths of your psycho-physical-spiritual self. These are not mindless mechanical "body-building" exercises. They are not your standard "I want to touch my toes." Who made up the obsession of touching your toes with straight legs? Why would you want to do that? Maybe for tying your shoes….

The EXploracises are a process that helps you touch something else: like curiosity, and the possibilities for changes in your being, including your animal, social, and divine selves. A transformational challenge. I am talking about the living body, the somatic element of life. Not simply feeling your body but feeling your organization and your synchronized embodiment of the moment.

As we continue to do the EX, let's use the ocean as a metaphor. The ocean has waves on top that we see. But there is more going on underneath, below the waves. The tide is coming in and going out. And beneath that is the current, flowing in a certain direction. I discovered this current when I moved to California, got my wetsuit, and jumped into the water. Little did I know about riptides! But it all ended well.

Take the ocean image into your body. Take a moment to recognize that we are interested in what goes on below the surface, like the ocean tides and currents. In ourselves we see what is happening "on top"—our behavior, gestures, and mannerisms, the cosmetic aspects—like the waves on the sea. But now we are also interested in what is going on inside, underneath the surface—the sensations, constrictions, flows, hidden emotions, and subtext. We want to go into the murky waters of shadow and trauma, as well as the waters of ecstatic joy and healing. Know that all the layers make up the whole synchronized embodied you.

Doing any EXploracise, some people will expand and feel wonderful, and others expand and feel awful. It depends on your history. With orienting, some feel great in the here and now. Others are terrified because trauma may have happened in the past, while they were in the here and now. An EXploracise can go in different directions for different people.

Do what you can. That said, there are biological programs, expectations—biological coherence. If I look and there is no tiger = I will be okay. If I look and there is a tiger = fight or flight or freeze. Past history changes the experience of now, so that even if there is no tiger, there may be a fight-or-flight reaction. Or if there is a tiger, maybe there will be no response. Everybody is different. I try to speak to the majority, but I am aware there are many variations. When doing EX, honor the internal messages. They are not random. They are your unique story. When you are doing an EX, listen closely, with reverence. Most people just push through. Body and mind recognize when you have had enough. Listen to small messages.

> "Our body is always trying to help us;
> respect what the body is trying to tell us."
>
> —*Dr. Stephen Porges*

II – SIMPLE MOVEMENT EXPLORACISES

EX – Three Choices

Check any area of your physicality. Is it rigid, braced, and hyper? Or flaccid, loose, and hypo? Or comfy in between? Try jaw, shoulders, or belly.

EX – Micro-movements (MM)

Exercise per se is not always necessary, but movement is. Small awakenings such as MM can stimulate blood flow and relieve constricted muscles. They can connect mind and body. And connect body to other body parts. This interrupts the holding or bracing cycle. If you tend to brace your shoulders, do small MM to alleviate the pressure.

EX – Hold Head

Hold your head in your hands. Hands on your forehead. Let your head rest in your hands. Feel the weight. After a few moments, you may find that you take a breath or sigh, and your head can feel more connected to your body.

EX – Thumb and Head

The base end of the thumb seems to be connected to the back base of the skull. Lay your hands on a table and notice the angle of the last joint (that is closest to your wrist) of your thumb. Is it pulled into your hand or freely coming out? Wiggle it a little. It feels like it connects to the lower, back side of your head. This can help relieve pressure at the base of your skull.

EX – Floating Shoulder

Move your shoulder till it floats. Especially up, to unburden your top ribs. It does not need to stay up, but it needs to be able to float up. Float in all directions: front, back, side, up, and down.

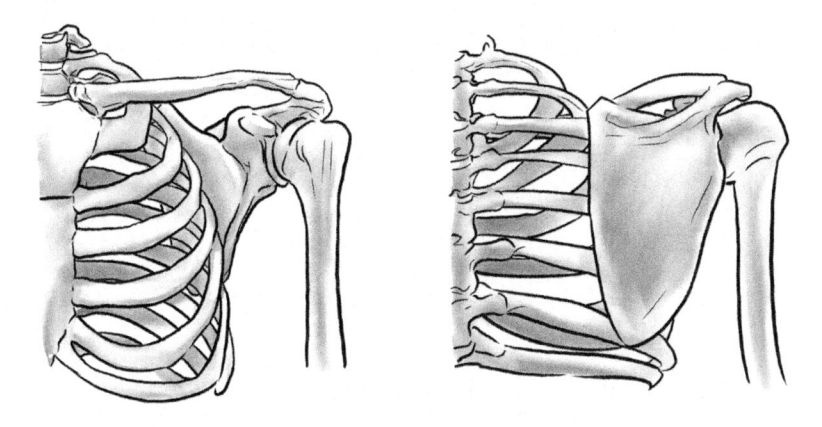

Shoulder

EX – Switch It

Many people have shoulders up and heart down, thereby feeling the startle pattern of shoulders pulled way up and the heart depressed down. We want to switch it to heart up and shoulders down.

A common "remedy" for this is to open your heart by pushing your chest out. This conceptualization is misinformed. It closes the back of your heart. This is not good. Hearts want to open in all directions—as does everything inside, an epic journey to your expanded self. Lungs fill, heart opens, ribs move, shoulders move. As your heart rises upward, your shoulders can drape downward.

EX – Five-Limb Flee

In a sitting position, push one foot into the ground, then the other, as if running in place. Bring in your hips. Bring in your shoulders. Bring in your arms. Allow your head to move. Breathe. Look around. Animals are four-limbed, five if you count the head. Allow all the limbs to be involved. Variation: You can do this starting with your head looking around. As you begin to run in place, add your arms and then legs. When you get to your feet, it adds a real thrust! And the power to get you to where you want to go.

II – SIMPLE MOVEMENT EXPLORACISES

EX – Dwell, or Bringing Attention to Bones
1, 2, 3, 4, 5

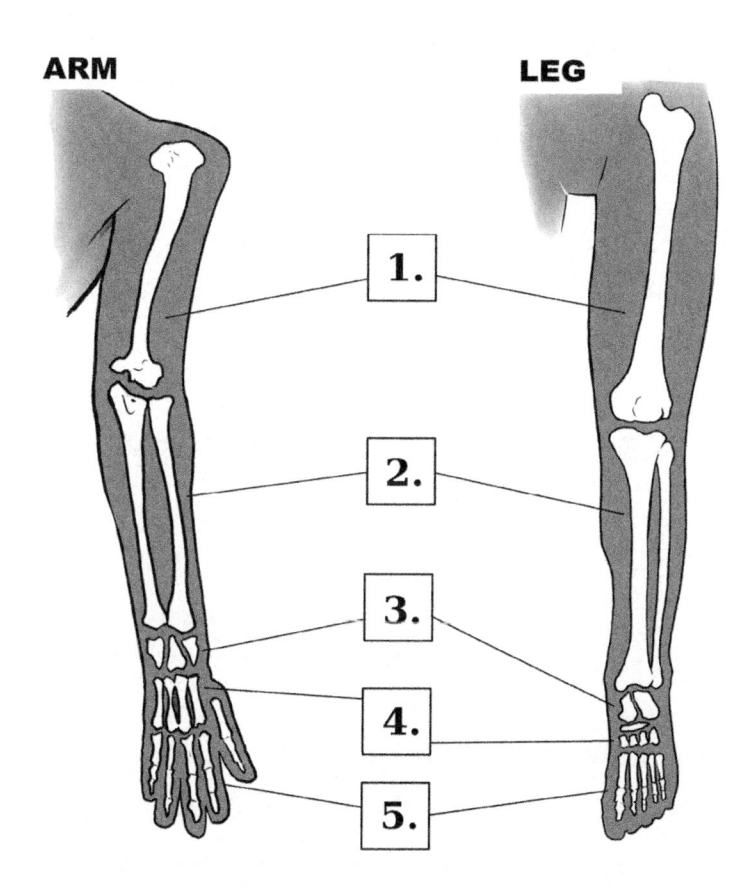

ARM **LEG**

1. Dwell in your upper arm.
2. Dwell in your lower arm.
3. Dwell in your wrist.
4. Dwell in your palm.
5. Dwell in your fingers.

EXPLORACISES

1. Dwell in your thigh.
2. Dwell in your lower leg.
3. Dwell in your ankle.
4. Dwell in your foot.
5. Dwell in your toes.

Dwell in your arms and legs together with an awareness of 1 through 5.

This 1,2,3,4,5, sequence is part of a kind of organization called sacred geometry. The body has numerical proportions of shapes and relationships. The proportion of head to body is usually one to seven. The arm span is similar to the body height. And recent research finds cells form sacred geometric proportional patterns in utero.[1]

EX – DNA Spirals

Lie down on your back, maybe in bed before sleep. Legs out straight.

1. Cross the right leg over, and cross the left arm over the body to hold the right shoulder. The leg that is crossed over makes a curve one way, and then the arm makes a curve the other way.
2. Reverse it. You will probably find that you have a preference for one combination or the other. Together, it looks like the DNA spiral.
3. You can also do this sitting. Cross your left leg over the right. And bring your right arm to your left shoulder. Stay there for a few moments. Then reverse it.
4. Physical contact with awareness allows for deep connection.

III – MULTILEVEL EXPLORACISES

EX – How You Think About Yourself

> "It all goes down in your mind."
>
> –*Johnny Cash*[2]

1. How do you think about yourself?
2. What do you imagine yourself to look like? Short, tall, fat, thin, a paper doll, a superhero?
3. Do you think of yourself as solid and heavy or porous and light?
4. Do you think about yourself as a divine light being having an earthly experience? Or an earthly being, just here doing whatever you do and getting by?
5. Do you think of your breath as a divine gift flowing through you from the Heavens? Or do you breathe just to stay alive and function, and hope for the best?

6. Do you move with such grace that the air moves around you and gently touches and bounces off your surroundings? Or do you move to get the job done, then finish and relax in front of the TV?
7. How you think about yourself influences your every move and your total environment.

EX – Lifting the Veil

PART 1

1. Start by exploring your peripheral vision.
2. Extend both hands in front of you at arm's length, fingers together.
3. Slowly open your fingers as you extend your arms out to your sides.
4. Let your eyes see as far as they can to the sides. In trauma we tend to narrow in on the danger and lose sight of the periphery.

PART 2

1. The cranial base of your head meets your spine behind your soft palate and between your ears. Your head moves from here, not the base of your neck. Often your head is pushing down, looking at a screen or emotionally pulled down.
2. Try moving your head slightly upward, like lifting a veil from your face with your hand. "Lifting the veil" is not a mechanical posture. Don't lift your head mechanically.
3. Feel the down of it, and allow the pull down to shift.

III – MULTILEVEL EXPLORACISES

4. Allow what is underneath to move upward. What happens to emotion, physicality, sensation, vibration, or image?
5. Explore PART 1 with your peripheral vision again after you lift the veil. Can you see further this time? Any more sense of poised uprightness?

EX – Head, Neck, and Shoulders: The Web Holds the Magic

So often I hear, "I hold so much tension in my shoulders and neck." This EX can help.

1. Start by gently stroking your head, neck, and shoulders. What do they feel like to you?
2. Gently move them. And feel the relationship between them.
3. Begin to move your arms: Push away, Hug, Embrace, Reach. What do your arms want to do?
4. Explore with your hands where your head meets your neck.
5. Explore with your hands where your neck meets your shoulders.
6. Your neck is a passageway. Is it open or closed?
7. Begin to slowly turn your head so that you add the spirals from your whole torso.
8. Spiral from your hips to your shoulder to the bottom of your skull, so that your head turns. What do you want to see? What do you not want to see? Right or left.
9. Now, allow your arms to move out from your back. Who do you want to push away? Who do you want to touch and hug? What or who do you want to reach for? Keep your legs involved.

10. Rest.
11. Are you tensing your shoulders and neck a bit less?
12. The web holds the magic. In other words, when you bring presence and movement to your head, neck, and shoulders, there is a wonderful web of amazing connection.

EX – Funny Bone Opens Heart

1. Sit or stand with your elbows pointing out to the side, and your hands resting on your shoulders.
2. Your "funny bone" is a nerve that runs along the outside of your elbow. It is the ulnar nerve. When it bangs or rubs up against your humerus (the bone in your upper arms), it creates the strange burning or tingling sensation from which it gets its name.
3. Feel your funny bone, with your upper arms parallel to the floor, and your hands near the side of your head. As you open your arms apart, you can feel your heart in the center. Your heart can open and lift. Twist side to side and feel your shoulder blades in the back connecting to your funny bone.
4. This can also be done with a group of three. One person on each side of you, holding your elbows.
5. Hold and support the elbow as you contact the funny bone.
6. Pull open to the side, and slightly up.
7. This movement lifts the heart like nothing else. It is related to reaching for love rather than protecting and pulling in.

III – MULTILEVEL EXPLORACISES

EX – Head Knuckle

1. Lie on your back. Bring your arms and hands up to your head.
2. Make a fist.
3. Place your fists in the groove of your temples.
4. Begin to move your head with your fists.
5. This helps to open the area under the arms. Armpits are a classic holding place. The fist helps move through any "fight" energy you may feel.
6. This leads to pedaling. One shoulder forward and one shoulder back with fists still on temples.
7. Start with shoulders pedaling backward, then forward.
8. Include your hips and whole body while still lying on your back.

EX – Trigeminal Leads to Oneness

The trigeminal is cranial nerve number 5 (CN V), one of the largest of the cranial nerves. The vagus is the longest, and the trigeminal is the widest. Its primary function is to provide sensory innervation to the different branches of the face, mainly the eyes and jaw. CN V seems to be a connector of body and head. Raymond Dart, the well-known Australian anatomist and anthropologist, wrote at length about the connecting and unifying properties of the trigeminal nerve.[3]

1. Lie down on your belly with your forehead on the floor, or you can do it on a bed. This engages the trigeminal nerve.
2. It may take a little adjusting to find a comfortable way to do this. Sometimes putting a pillow under your chest can help. If you need to, invent a holding device to be on your belly.

3. This position engages an inner spiral that connects and makes a pathway from your head to your torso. Having your trigeminal engaged is the opposite of a startle pattern with your head pulled back and down.
4. Try it standing: trigeminal on the wall. Stand at an even wall, facing the wall. Toes touch the wall, with weight on your heels.
5. Now explore three positions.
6. Put your chin on the wall = this disconnects your head from your body. It is basically a shutdown position.
7. Put your nose on the wall = sympathetic pattern of surprise or shock.
8. Put your upper forehead or hairline on the wall = trigeminal nerve engaged with ventral vagal connection.
9. As your forehead and inner head spiral forward, your lower back and bottom ribs widen.
10. Step away. Walk with this. You can put your hand on your forehead as a reminder.

EX – Be in Your Own Back while Sitting

We are very frontal beings. For the most part, we look forward, we speak forward, and we move forward. But we know cognitively that we are three-dimensional beings, with a front, two sides, and a back. These days with so much attention given to screens, cameras, and frontal interaction, it is easy to forget you have a back. Remember the phrases "I have your back," "She has a strong backbone," "The backbone of society."

III – MULTILEVEL EXPLORACISES

1. Sit in a chair and bring your awareness to your feet on the floor.
2. As you sense the solidity of the ground, let the ground support you, as your leg muscles engage.
3. Your sitting bones on the chair parallel your feet on the ground. They connect, and they receive support from the chair.
4. This support travels up your back, filling your back. You fill your back like you would stuff a pillow with feathers, gently adding more support until you feel the fullness. Recognize the length and width of your back, along with the gentle curves of your spine. This brings attention to space, mobility, and strength.
5. The width wants to be felt all the way up and down your spine. At the base, around your pelvis, it can feel like your pants pockets stretching apart. At your lower ribs, you can imagine a smile across your mid-back. In your upper back, you can feel your shoulder blades gliding apart. Your spine travels upward behind your tongue and mouth. And as the top of your spine meets your cranial base, feel your middle ears moving away from each other.
6. Notice how all of this breathes.
7. Your 3D torso includes your 3D breath. Touch and connect them with your hands or your imagination.
8. Next time you sit at a computer or talk to someone, feel what it's like to be in your own back.

EXPLORACISES

EX – Bicycle Sitting

1. Sit on a chair, legs apart. Lean forward and then return to center, pivoting from your hips. Lean your elbows on your thighs the whole time. Find a rhythm.
2. Lean forward and back. Add one shoulder rolling forward. Right shoulder forward as you move forward, right shoulder back as you move back. Left shoulder forward as you move forward, left shoulder back as you move back.
3. Bring the right shoulder halfway to the left knee as you move forward. Bring the left shoulder halfway to the right knee as you move forward.
4. Add right shoulder rolls rotating in a circle as you move forward toward the knee. The shoulder will roll forward as you lean forward, and it will roll back as you lean back. Same with the left.
5. One heel at a time comes up. The heel comes up as you move back. The right shoulder rolls back as the right heel comes up. Then the left shoulder rolls back as the left heel comes up.
6. It feels like you are bicycling with a twist in your torso.
7. Allow your head to turn.
8. Go as far as you can go in each direction.
9. Added notes: Lean your elbows on your thighs the whole time. Let the arms extend and move from the shoulders. Let the arms reach as far as they can reach with the elbows on the thighs. Left arm forward, right arm back, head looking right.

III – MULTILEVEL EXPLORACISES

EX – Infinity: Ripple 8s

Lying down or standing up, start by making circles with your shoulders and hips. There are diagonal cross lines connecting your shoulders and hips.

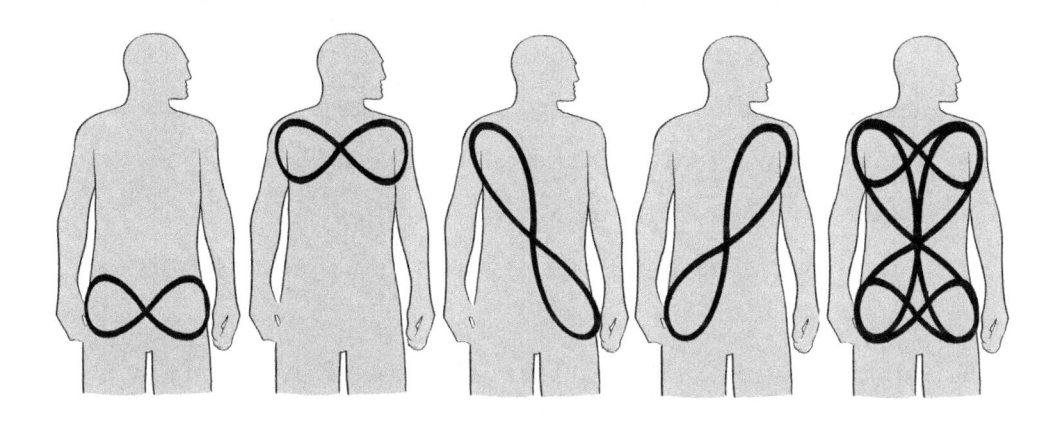

Figure 8

1. Do a simple twist to feel and connect. Stabilize the hips and move a shoulder forward and backward, one side at a time. Reverse. Stabilize your shoulders and move your hip forward and backward, one side at a time.
2. Forward and back
   Stabilize hips and move shoulders: right shoulder forward and left shoulder back. Then reverse.
   Stabilize shoulders and move hips: right hip forward and left hip back. Then reverse.
3. Up and down
   Now it's the same position but moving up and down.
   Stabilize hips and move shoulders: right shoulder up and left

shoulder down. Reverse.

Stabilize shoulders and move hips: right hip up and left hip down. Reverse.

4. Combine: do forward-and-back movements together, hips and shoulders in opposition. Right hip forward, left shoulder back. Left hip forward, right shoulder back.
5. Combine up and down: right hip up and right shoulder up. Do left. Connect belly and heart.
6. Make a horizontal figure 8 with both shoulders.
7. Make a horizontal figure 8 with your hips.
8. Add forward, back, up, and down to your figure 8s in shoulders and hips.
9. Do the figure 8 in hips and shoulders together, up and down and forward and back.
10. All together and let head and arms and legs ripple.
11. If this is confusing, don't worry, just make any kind of figure 8 with your shoulders and hips.
12. The figure 8 or sign of infinity has been used by many Indigenous peoples for healing and connecting to higher energies. You can walk in a figure 8 or move the figure 8 around or within your body. Hope Fitzgerald teaches "The Infinity Wave."

EX – Lengthen the Lower Back

1. Lie down with your knees bent and feet flat. When trying to lengthen the lower back, most people just lift their hips. This jams your hip joints and does not allow maximum length. Try this:

2. As you do your lying-down work, pay attention to your breath, and on your exhale let your pelvis drop to the floor (not forced).
3. Let your heels drop into the floor a bit more actively.
4. Let them drop in more and let the bottom of your pelvis lift up a bit. Allow your pelvic floor to open to this, as your lower back lengthens.

EX – Molding Palms

Our own hands have a wonderful healing quality. Placing your palms on yourself in areas that your hands easily mold to is one way to experience this. You may need to wiggle around a bit to find a good fit, either a suction or a sealed contact. Try the areas listed and find more of your own! Other body parts and combinations not listed here mold to each other.

1. Palm on cheekbone.
2. Palm over eyes.
3. Palm on bottom skull in back.
4. Palm on jawbone horizontally in front.
5. Palms on top shoulders.
6. Palms on front bottom ribs.
7. Palms on side ribs—thumbs on bottom ribs.
8. Palms on hip crest—thumb inside.
9. Palms on sides of hips with thumbs on hip socket.
10. One foot on top of the other at the arches.
11. Toes on toes.
12. Bend knees on top of each other.

13. Palm on ankle, where foot meets lower leg. Fingers hook at ankle.
14. If your life allows it, "spoon" with another person.

EX – Habits

Stand in a space where you have room to walk.

1. Start with your feet together. Begin to walk forward. Notice which foot steps first. Stop after four or five steps. Feet together and repeat (3X). Which foot led?
2. Start with your feet together. Begin to walk forward, but this time lead with your habitually nondominant foot (3X).
3. You are out of your habit. You may wonder why you always lead with one foot or why you never lead with the other one. WHY do we do this simple exploration? At some point in your healing, as the somatic pattern shifts, you will experience some change in yourself. It will be unfamiliar and feel weird, odd, or different. Your sense of self changes. This walking EX can give a taste of how it may feel to be out of your habitual mode. Remember that this is just "me" out of my habitual pattern.

III – MULTILEVEL EXPLORACISES

EX – Bracing Pattern in Motion

1. Start to walk around the room.
2. Stop and notice how you stop.
3. Explore the two main choices:
4. You can contract all your muscles to stop yourself. Or…
5. You can just stop walking.
6. Notice that 4 stresses the system more and continues to reinforce the bracing patterns, and 5 begins to release the system.

EX – Shift Weight Standing

1. Full-body movements stimulate the baroreceptors, the blood-pressure feedback loops.
2. Shift weight from foot to foot.
3. Find the moment you are crossing from one foot to the other.
4. Where is that weight change in your physicality?
5. Where is there no weight on either foot?
6. Take a walk with that.

EX – Inside Touch

PART 1

1. Notice any difficult emotion(s) that you might have.
2. Notice what happens when you think about this. Shame, unworthiness, and self-criticism often have a collapsed or dropped-down aspect.
3. For a moment let yourself feel what it might be like for that to change.
4. Remember that under your skin is a layer of fascia that creates an elastic encasement, an elastic envelope.
5. Allow the difficult emotion to be touched from inside by the three-dimensional web of the fascial matrix.
6. Perhaps make a move slightly upward, from inside, to free away from the drop down. A moment of fluidity.

PART 2

1. Think of a moment of overwhelm, with a physical fall or a shoulder bump, when the elastic suit was breached, or the border was broken or compromised.
2. Don't go inside the crack from the outside. Stay at the spot of impact with inside touch.
3. Renew the flow of the elastic envelope in your whole body, as you allow healing to occur from the inside.

III – MULTILEVEL EXPLORACISES

EX – Outside Touch

From the moment we are conceived, we are touching. The actual sense of touch develops in the sixth week of embryonic life and encompasses all our systems. There are so many variations of touch, some welcome, some not. Baby mammals that do not receive nurturing touch tend to not thrive. How you give and receive touch can be a lifelong exploration. You may want your intimate partner to touch you, but if the touch is not sensitive to your needs, it may be unpleasant. The contact immediately stirs up a psychological response. Dr. Aline LaPierre has coined the term "NeuroAffective Touch, the gentle art of blending psychotherapeutic skill with the therapeutic use of attuned touch."[4] Let's explore some touch.

PART 1

1. Often, when somebody says something about themselves, like, *"Oh, I'm sorry,"* they bring their hand up to their heart. Place your hand on your own heart. Stay there for a few moments. Feel the contact of your hand. What do you feel? Softness? Warmth? Pressure? Nothing?

PART 2

1. Touch helps you contain your feelings and emotions, and it supports you holding new thoughts, sensations, and responses. Place your hand on your opposite upper arm. Right hand on left upper arm.
2. Touch your skin boundary to contain. Hold with compassion for what happened or didn't happen.

3. Squeeze deeper to feel your muscles. Both being touched and touching. Notice breath. If your arm is numb, send an invitation: *You can come back now. Tell me your story.*
4. Release the pressure and feel the effect on your whole arm or upper body.
5. Move your hand to your lower upper arm and repeat the sequence.
6. Do the other side. Left hand on right upper arm.

Often, the tightness is a defense pattern. Do you still need the holding to be this present or this strong? The answer may be yes or no, as you return to yourself and inquire within.

EX – Pick Me Up

1. Under your arm about six inches down on the side of your torso, three muscles gather. The latissimus dorsi comes down from your armpit and goes to your back. The serratus is in the center. The oblique crosses in front of your torso. They gather at a spot under your arm on the side. A tiny nerve gathers them together. I learned this anatomical fact from Gil Hedley, the wonderful anatomist.[5] Then I explored:
2. Cross your arms and hold yourself there.
3. This is where we would be picked up from, as a baby or child.
4. Feel like you are getting picked up. Or you are wanting to be picked up. Who picked you up? Who did you want to pick you up?
5. Add a slight lift with your hands in that area.
6. Now we pick ourselves up.

III – MULTILEVEL EXPLORACISES

> "Pick yourself up, dust yourself off,
> and start all over again."
>
> —*Dorothy Fields*

EX – Crack Open

1. Find one place that needs a little extra attention now—maybe a point of constriction or trembling, or it's shaky or buzzy.
2. Stay with it. Be with it. Is there any sensation, image, color, movement, or texture?
3. Do *Humm* to it. (Chapter 3, EX – HUMM 1)
4. As you stay with it, is there any small crack, flow, or change?
5. Use that opening to receive a change or shift. A crack to let the light in.
6. Don't look for a huge breakthrough and be disappointed if it does not happen, but instead allow time and space for something just a bit different to show up, a new response or interest.

> "Light will someday split you open,
> even if your life is now a cage."
>
> —*Hafiz, Persian poet and mystic*

EXPLORACISES

EX – Rumi: Open/Close Fist

> "Your hand opens and closes, opens and closes. If it were always a fist or always stretched open, you would be paralyzed. Your deepest presence is in every small contracting and expanding, the two as beautifully balanced and coordinated as birds' wings."
>
> —*Rumi*

Expansion and contraction are the movements of the universe in all aspects, including our nervous system's charge/discharge, excite/settle.

1. Look at expansion and contraction in your hands. Make a fist, then open your hand, then close, etc.
2. As you continue to open and close your hands, first look at your hands, then feel them, then feel your body, then notice emotion. You may observe yourself as receptive, vulnerable, powerful, strong, or hiding.
3. This is a way to start paying attention to your body, if that is unfamiliar for you, or this also can be used to slow down.
4. Cycles can happen. At some point the contraction releases to expansion; then the expansion folds into contraction.
5. Our natural rhythm can get lost. We lose our groove. We each have a vibration and a rhythm. When we interfere with that, we lose access to our authentic self. Look for your natural rhythm as you start to move your whole body with your hands' expansion and contraction. If you are alive, there is rhythm and movement

III – MULTILEVEL EXPLORACISES

somewhere. Explore this. The rhythm of your authentic self reveals your wholeness.

6. Rest.
7. Bring your hands up to face each other. Let your hands have a conversation. Let them speak about how they feel. Are they different or similar?
8. Explore the energy between your hands, as they move apart and together. Let your hands come together at the end. They find oneness: "the two as beautifully balanced and coordinated as birds' wings."

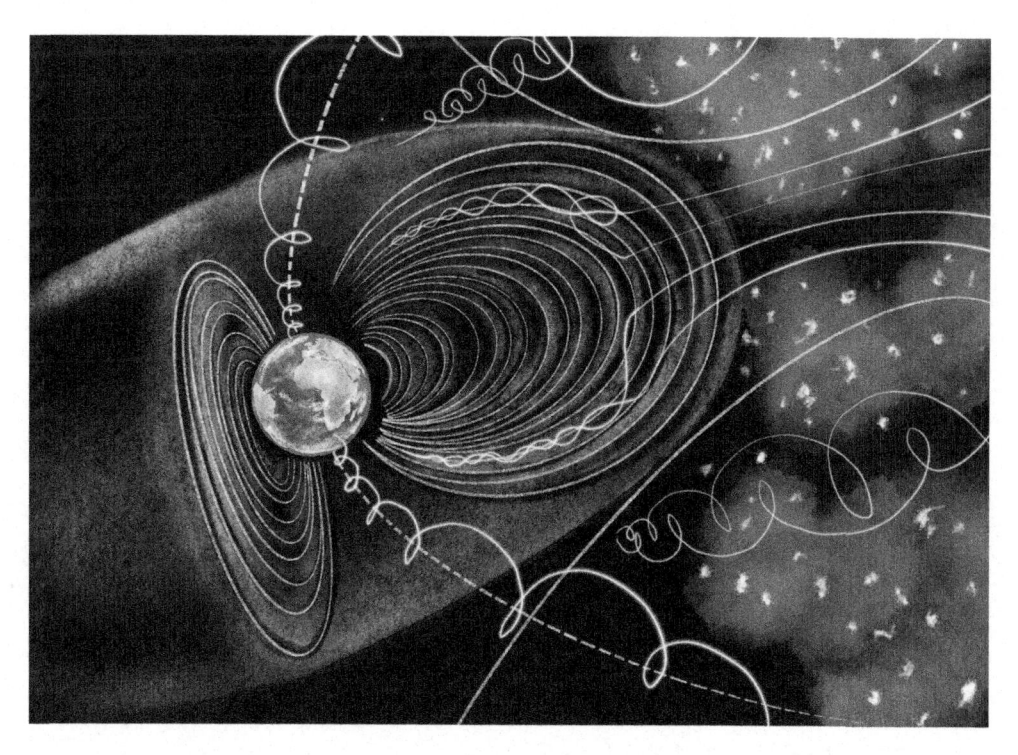

Earth's pulsating magnetic field

EXPLORACISES

EX – Need to Let Go vs. Let Go the Need

There is a common phrase in healing today, "Let go" (of this holding or that habit). But letting go is not what really happens on the physical level. As we saw with our fascia, we are one 3D entity, so there is no letting go of one part without affecting the whole. Many of the holdings were established unconsciously as survival patterns; you cannot just let go a muscle and think you have solved the issue. Patterns develop because of a need that is physical, mental, and emotional. Don't let go—understand the need. For example:

1. You might always be helping friends… perhaps in a way that is not totally genuine. But you need to help them. When you realize that you need to help to feel worthy, you are able to explore why you do not feel worthy, and the compulsive helping can subside.
2. Define your needs and see what needs can be met in a different way.
3. Don't "let go" of your shallow breathing. Find the need for your limited breath. Breathe and notice and don't try to change. But it will change. As soon as you bring attention to it, it will change. This process is not manipulating yourself as if you were an object. But breath changes according to what you are doing. If I walk, I breathe. If I run, I breathe faster. There is a different breathing tempo if I am thinking about something, past or future, or if I am here now watching how I breathe in the present moment, and understanding my needs.

III – MULTILEVEL EXPLORACISES

EX – Change

1. What is present for you now, as a result of doing the EXploracises?
2. What has changed? Relationships? Bracing patterns? Finished or started a project, or maybe an inner change? Let's explore.
3. If you have two chairs nearby, use them. If not, just angle yourself in your chair in two different directions.
4. Physical: First chair. When I started the EXploracises, I ____ (could never feel supported. Or I noticed tightening or collapse in my body, mind, and emotion). Fill in the blanks with your experiences.
   Second chair. Today, I am here, and I ____ (felt supported a couple of times. Or My body is stronger, and I am more stable).
5. Emotional: First chair. When I started the EXploracises, I ____ (felt angry and anxious quite often. Or I felt everybody was more important than me).
   Second chair. Today, I am here, and I ____ (have moments of feeling calmer, and I am able to understand my anger more, while having more compassion for myself).
6. Spiritual: First chair. When I started the EXploracises, I ____ (felt myself mechanistic and robot-like as I went through my day).
   Second chair. Today, I am here, and I ____ (have moments of feeling like I have more flow as I move through my day. And I am willing to explore that I am a divine being having an earthly experience).

EXPLORACISES

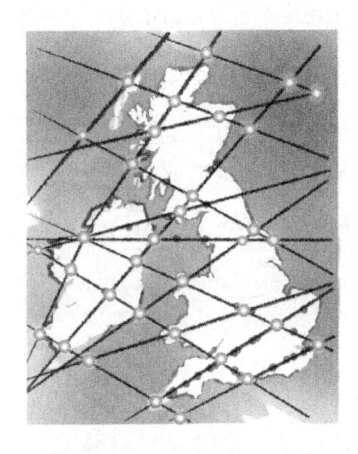

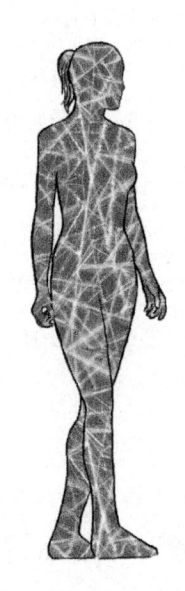

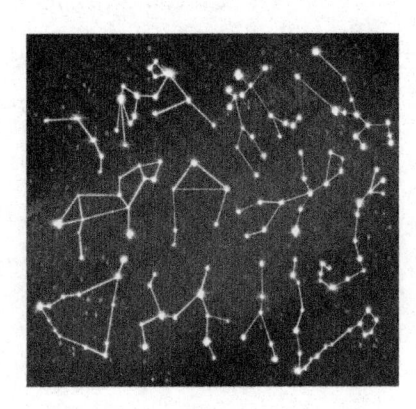

Ley lines, fascia, cosmos

CHAPTER 5

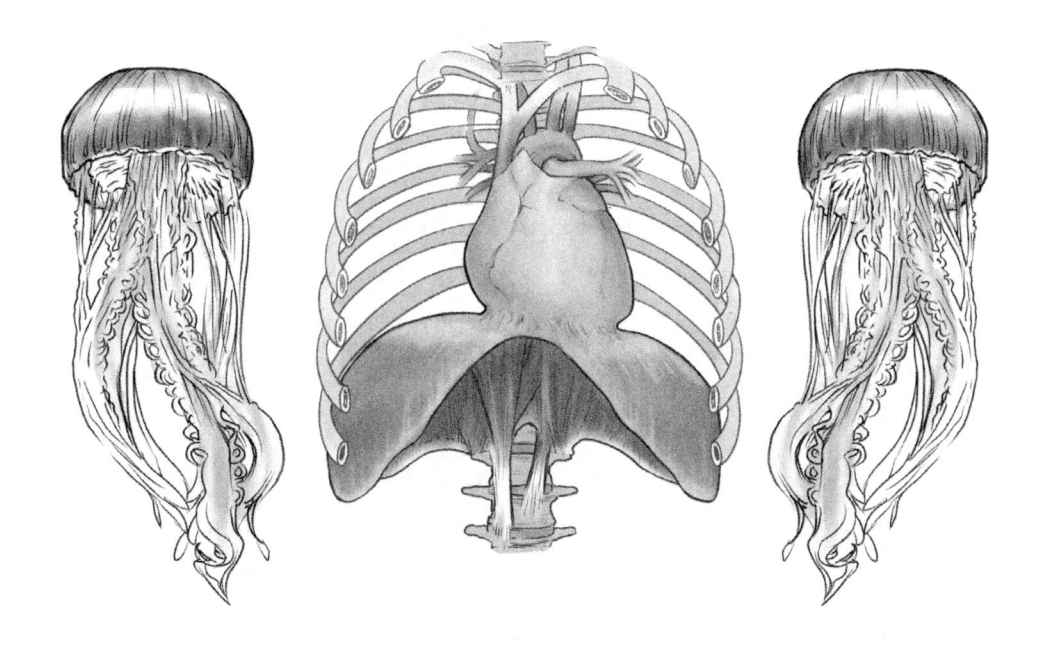

BREATH

I – INTRODUCTION TO BREATH

Breath is freely given. Air flows in and out as seamlessly as the rain falls, without notice or effort. Breath is a strong wind or a gentle breeze, depending on the outer activity and inner thoughts, feelings, ideas, and perceptions. There are certain anatomical facts about how the respiratory system functions optimally. There is also the reality of how emotions tell you that you need to breathe or not breathe now. You can be fascinated with both. You can stay with the way you breathe, or you can try on many different breathing explorations. Living organisms on our planet have been breathing for billions of years. As you bathe in the awareness of breath, the power of life from the Heavens and Earth emerges.

I – INTRODUCTION TO BREATH

EX – Breath Choice

1. You can choose to stay with your well-worn adaptive pattern.
2. Or you can choose to join the universally designed organization created eons ago in a faraway cosmos. The universe affects the atmospheric pressure, which affects us. This breath that allows minimum effort and maximum efficiency is explained in the following EXs.

For young children, there is not always an open pathway for emotions to flow out. The well-warranted anger has no outlet. Thus, it gets held inside, often, with restricted breath. Blocked breath holds valuable information. We all have exiles, parts of ourselves that we needed to hide away. How do exiles breathe? Emotions are masked or hidden in breath. The place where there is limited breath holds secrets that are waiting to be revealed. A gentle, respectful approach is suggested.

Many popular styles of breathing therapy these days are aggressive and showy—methods that produce large physical and emotional changes. But do they train enough subtlety for our human system? Too many people are learning to push their breath and manipulate their bodies without changing the deep subtle emotions and long-held patterns that cause the constrictions they are manipulating.

EXPLORACISES

EX – Breath in the Moment

I am interested in what is happening to the individual in the moment and the influence of stored behaviors, emotions, and traumas.

1. Changes in these realms are possible as you begin to pay attention to structure, flow, function, and reality.
2. Can you recognize where the interference is to your breath?
3. Can you arrive at this with your own awareness?
4. When you feel your own restrictions, you are up against your own resistance.
5. Your restrictions point to where the interference may have begun. When it began may have been a traumatic incident.
6. If you layer forced breath on top of old breath, on top of dysfunctional patterns of breath, what gain have you made?

It may be a better idea to teach functional breathing for everyday use instead of Olympic breathing for competing. This healthier approach is to invite body, mind, and spirit to welcome whatever breath comes in to replenish the oxygen. Then follow your exhale to the natural conclusion, a fuller exhale. Extending your exhale, not manipulating, can be a way to reduce pain, emotional or physical. We want to get rid of excess carbon dioxide and also build some tolerance to let the carbon dioxide do its valuable jobs, including transporting hemoglobin.

The natural sensors in your brain will regulate breath. The phrenic nerve sensor says when it is time to breathe, which is when you have too much carbon dioxide, not when you need oxygen. If your ribs are not held too tightly, they will release to create a vacuum, and breath will flow in like opening a window on a spring day. The miracle of the breath is that various techniques change people's awareness of breath,

1 – INTRODUCTION TO BREATH

so that it is an invitation through physical changes to access higher states of consciousness.

Look around—no matter where you are, alone or with people, on screen or in person—and notice that everybody is breathing, in and out. Everybody has deep feelings inside, some painful, some less so. Breathe. Your breath is not something that you do but rather a response to what you are doing, thinking, and imagining. You think of some past trauma and you will breathe one way with your whole body. Then you experience the change or healing that can take place, and you breathe another way. Breath is both a response to trauma (constriction) and a resource for health (expansion). And your breath is helping you realize or is telling you that there will always be in and out, expansion and contraction, both with deep feelings. And no matter how deep or painful your feelings or wounds are, some healing or wholeness can occur. We want to hold space for that embodied synchronicity.

A student was talking about his breath. He said "the" breath. I said to him, "It is 'your' breath."

He said, "It is 'our' breath."

II – BREATHING EXPLORACISES

EX – Optimal Breath

If I hear someone audibly breathe in, on a podcast, during a lecture, or in casual conversation, I know the respiratory mechanism is not working optimally. Most people, if asked to take a "deep breath," will proceed to suck air into their lungs to puff up their front chest. This is far from optimal.

1. According to our functional structure, when you allow the proper expansion of the chest (also called the thorax), this creates a vacuum.
2. This vacuum causes the nostrils to be dilated and the lungs to be instantly and quietly filled with air by atmospheric pressure. So much less effort. A spontaneous breath.
3. You never have to "take" a breath again or gasp for an inhale. Breath is reflexive.

II – BREATHING EXPLORACISES

4. Stop holding your ribs so tightly that they cannot allow the chest expansion. Of course, this is not so easy given the emotional holding that most of us have in the muscular and fascial lining of our chest, which affects the elastic system of the whole body.

5. It is possible to be breathing by a beautifully poised and automatic dynamic balance between pressure differences in your chest cavity and the entire atmosphere of the Earth, and the elasticity of your ribs and lungs and associated respiratory organs. Expansion and contraction, alternately.

6. Respiratory education needs to include the principles of atmospheric pressure, the equilibrium of the whole body, and the alternate expansions and contractions of the thorax or ribcage. The atmospheric pressure, which is about fifteen pounds per square inch on the surface of the Earth, actively pushes air into our nose and/or mouth when we create a vacuum by expanding our ribcage and lowering our diaphragm. That is all that is necessary for air to come rushing into our thorax. No need at all to effort and suck air in.

7. The key here is training a well-functioning thoracic mechanism, securing the maximum thoracic mobility and expansion while preventing thoracic rigidity. For optimal breath, these expansions increase the capacity of the chest that is necessary to facilitate the normal oscillations of atmospheric pressure. This natural action ensures that the throat and neck muscles, as well as the larynx and the shoulders, remain passive; the breath will pass noiselessly into the lungs, while those passages will dilate instead of contract. (Most people constrict their nostrils to pull in a breath.) With this absolute control and freedom of

the thoracic mechanism, you can secure an adequate air supply through the nostrils while singing, speaking, sleeping, or exerting physical effort. I hope this explanation makes it clearer why "belly breathing" is not optimal.

EX – Breathing Tips

- No part of your diaphragm is below your ribs. So, do not put your hand on your belly and tell me you are touching your diaphragm.
- Since your diaphragm is involved whenever you breathe, all breathing can be called diaphragmatic breathing.
- The apex or top of your lungs is a quarter of an inch above your collarbone.

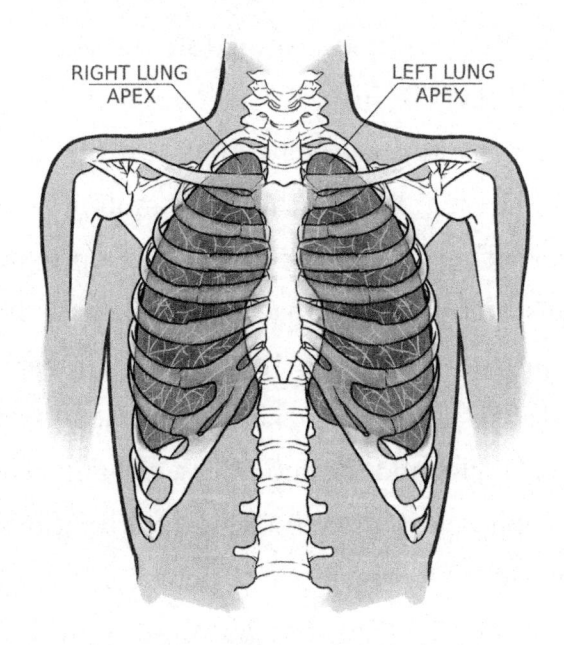

Lungs

11 – BREATHING EXPLORACISES

- Nose breathing is more efficient than mouth breathing for everyday breathing.
- The nose orchestrates innumerable functions in our body to keep us balanced.
- We take 25,000 breaths a day.
- If you are having a panic attack, do not take a deep breath. Slow, light breath is better.
- For stress, breathing out with a sigh can be helpful. Neurons control the sigh, and it signals relaxation.
- A monastic practice: Quiet your breath so that a feather under your nose does not move when you breathe.
- Breath is the behind-the-scenes controller. It is voluntary and involuntary, conscious and subconscious. Because it is conscious and subconscious, it may be the link between the two.
- If you close your eyes to breathe, let your eyes move as you breathe. Do not fix them.
- Air comes into the lungs in a spiral formation.

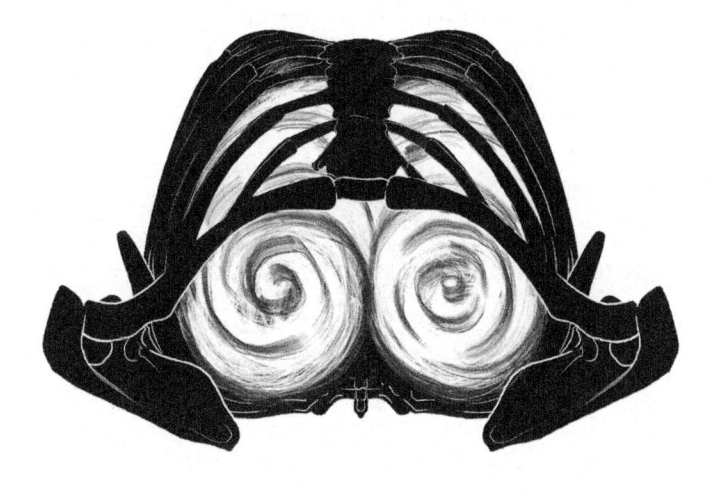

Smoke spiraling in the lungs

EXPLORACISES

EX – Let's Look at Three Aspects of Breath

1. With fear and anxiety, your breath can speed up or slow down. Watch how fast breath comes in and goes out. With awareness, this speed may shift.
2. Rest. Notice where there is movement or not, when you are generally breathing. Shape changes happen. What is moving or not moving? Place your hands on the side of your ribs: when one area moves, what happens to the area next to it? Does the movement, space, or expansion spread? Notice that you are not getting rid of anything. You are becoming aware.
3. Are any emotions showing up for you that were hidden or blocked by held breath? Are those emotions tucked away to not feel the fear, sadness or anger, compassion or empathy for other or self? Just notice.

You will be noticing these three elements (speed of breath, movement in the body related to breath, and surfacing emotions) in all the following EX. All the explorations I am presenting are intended to help you discover what you are doing with your breath, and ideally to regulate it better if necessary. We are not getting rid of anything or denying any emotions. We are exploring what happens when you bring awareness to breathing. Regulating can allow you to hold more oxygen, enables you to pass more easily through stressful states, and has other health benefits.

II – BREATHING EXPLORACISES

EX – Breath and Shoulders

1. Breathing moves your whole physicality, both what is on the surface and what is deep inside.
2. Notice your breath. Eyes open or closed is fine.
3. Do not do anything to try to change your breath or your posture. No need to try for a longer inhale or exhale. You are not trying to fix, heal, or understand. Now it is okay to just notice.
4. No need to make it better. One way is not better than another, right now. We want to accept breath as it is. We are simply interested in what is....
5. The rhythm of the breath can change moment to moment. Allow the change. Continue watching breath come in and go out.
6. Notice your shoulders. As you breathe, your shoulders respond to your lungs filling, and they want to move on your ribcage. They move from the bottom because your ribs push them. They do not move from the top of your shoulders. They are not lifted from above.
7. When you breathe in or out, are you holding your shoulders, front and back?
8. Even if you do cadence or 5-5 breathing (presented later in this chapter), if your shoulders are braced or your neck is tight, you will not get the full benefit of it.
9. Shoulders are made to slide and glide on your back as you breathe.

EX – Breathe Through Your Nose

1. Your nose has one main function, and that is for you to breathe. If possible, use it for that. Some people have obstructions in their nose that force them to mouth-breathe.
2. Your nose filters, warms, and purifies the raw air.
3. When you inhale through your nose, the breath gently sweeps across the pituitary, the master hormonal gland. This can trigger different hormones to flood into your body. It can lower your blood pressure, monitor heart rate, and help store memories.
4. You can tape your mouth closed when you sleep to encourage your nose to do its job. This has been shown to reduce snoring and sore throats. If there has been any kind of oral trauma, this practice may not be the best option.
5. All that said about the benefits of nose breathing, I am aware that there are many styles of breathing that involve mouth breathing that induce different states of consciousness or body awareness.

EX – Nitric Oxide

1. Nitric oxide is produced in nasal passages as part of the defense system against bacterial and viral infections.
2. Breathing through your nose increases nitric oxide.
3. Nitric oxide opens up blood vessels and widens capillaries, called *vasodilation,* meaning it relaxes the smooth inner muscles of the blood vessels, causing them to dilate and increase circulation. This increases oxygen intake.

II – BREATHING EXPLORACISES

EX – Humming

1. Humming while exhaling instantly increases the nitric oxide concentration in the nasal passages and sinuses, sometimes producing fifteen times more nitric oxide.
2. Research shows that humming reduces stress, invites calmness, and encourages sleep. It lowers heart rate and blood pressure and produces powerful neurochemicals such as oxytocin, the "love" hormone.
3. Hum your favorite song.

EX – Breathing Trio

Like a musical trio, each participant plays their part, and they all play together.

1. Start with both hands opening and closing with your breath. Close on exhale. Open on inhale. Do the exhale first. Find your rhythm.
2. Continue opening and closing your hands, as you place them on the sides of your head. Touching the head is the "close" part; moving them slightly away is the "open" part. Breathe and notice what happens in your brain.
3. With the same motion, place both hands on your heart. Breathe and notice what happens in your heart.
4. With the same motion, place both hands on your belly. Breathe and notice what happens in your belly.
5. Move your hands around and try different combinations.
6. Notice all three moving together (head, heart, belly) with or without your hand contact.

EXPLORACISES

EX – Diaphragm Dancing Orchestra

The whole diaphragm is like a musical instrument that wants to be ready to move and/or play at all times. If one part is stuck, the vibrations do not transmit to the surrounding muscles, organs, tissues, etc. The music is not complete and stagnation sets in. Often unnoticed for a while, the non-movement prevents blood flow and healthy breathing. And long-term consequences are certain to show up.

1. Interlock your fingers to make a dome shape, like your diaphragm.
2. Move them up and down.
3. Down for the inhale. And up for the exhale.
4. Watch your diaphragm from inside, rising and falling. It rises on your exhale and drops down and out on your inhale.

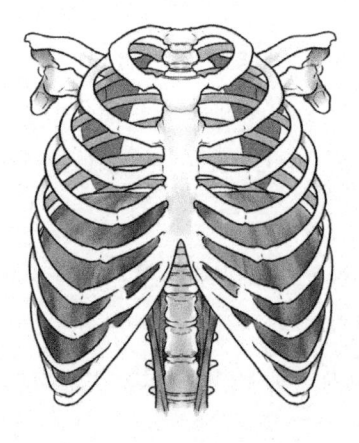

EXHALE   INHALE

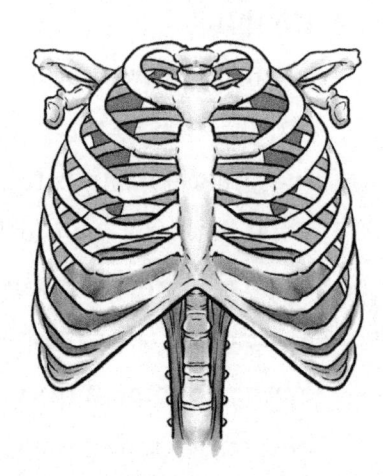

Diaphragm

II – BREATHING EXPLORACISES

EX – The Breath and Rib Reset

1. Put your hands on your bottom ribs on both sides.
2. Slightly push in the bottom flared rib—push it in a little more than it is used to at the end of your exhale.
3. Hold it a few seconds.
4. Recognize that the brain is first disorganized and confused (this is not what we always do, or this is not my habit).
5. Stop the pressure and let the rib spring back out for the inhale.
6. The brain will search for a readjustment: how can I find my way to a new breath?
7. Settling in a slightly new place, your breath is a little deeper and a little more elastic. Let your breath adjust and repeat (3X).

EX – Springiness of Ribs

The manubrium is the wide upper part of your sternum (breast bone). It has cartilage joints connected to your first and second ribs. These joints often have a raised ridge, with a hardness or constriction, which affects your shoulders, jaw, upper chest, head angle, and more.

1. To find this joint while lying down, palpate your collarbone from your shoulder to the center of your torso. You come to an edge, you feel a hole, drop into it. From the top of your sternum, go down one inch to find your manubrium.

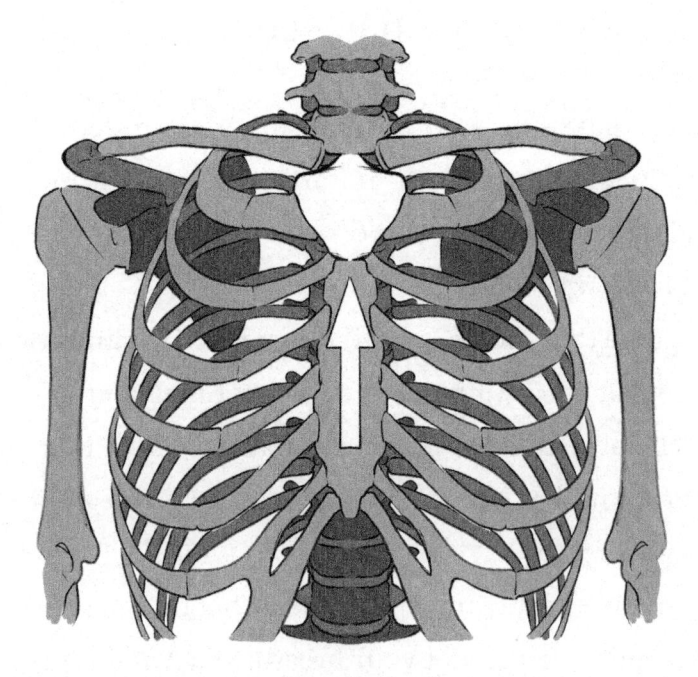

Manubrium

2. Gently explore the movability, as you press the manubrium to the floor or toward the spine. When you can allow it to spring back, you have a spontaneous breath.
3. With this, your back can open and widen across your shoulders.
4. Move down your sternum and gently push each rib's attachment on both sides of your sternum. And let them spring up. Inspiration!
5. Get to the bottom of the sternum.
6. Continue and touch around your lower ribs till you get to the lowest place, where ribs meet hip crests at your sides. This helps access back rib movement.
7. Move the bottom ribs to access the elasticity of the diaphragm. A healthy system is multidimensionally springy.

EX – Variation, starting at the bottom:

1. Place your hands on the sides of your chest, with your fingertips on your side ribs, and your thumbs on your back bottom ribs.
2. As you exhale, press the ribs gently down.
3. See if you can find the spring up that allows the spontaneous breath.
4. The spine does not collapse. It continues to aim up.
5. Starting at your bottom ribs on the side, go up each rib, pushing and releasing, ending up in your armpit. It probably hurts in your armpit, as it is often very tender.
6. Alternate side to side. One hand at a time.
7. This often increases breath in the upper chest. Very good to get breath moving!
8. Your chest becomes a treasure chest with gold oxygen inside.

EX – The Two Nostrils Are Different

1. You want to balance your system.
2. Block one nostril and breathe through the other.
3. Right nostril breath: Circulation speeds up, gets hot; cortisol and blood pressure increase. Your right nostril affects the left side of your brain.
4. Left nostril breath: Circulation slows down, gets cooler; blood pressure decreases. Your left nostril activates the right side of your brain.

You can see why you want to breathe through your nose if possible. Your mouth cannot do anything like this. It can't balance your system.

EX – Emotion and Breath

I was feeling a bit angry and tired. I realized my right nostril was not as free as it could be. I blocked my left nostril and encouraged my right to do something different. At first it was not budging. I almost could not breathe. But after a while, it opened, and something moved through. Coincidentally, my anger diminished. Our breath reflects our emotions.

1. When you are crying, your breath is very heavy and pressured.
2. When you feel joy, your breath can be light and buoyant.
3. Changing your breath can change emotion.

EX – Breath: Exhale 1

1. When you notice that you are not breathing, the first instinct is to try to inhale for more breath.
2. But let's look at what might be going on.
3. Most people do not exhale fully. There are many reasons for this, with anxiety among them, causing breath to be high in the chest.
4. Because of the incomplete exhales, carbon dioxide gets stuck or trapped in the lungs, giving a feeling of needing more oxygen.
5. Then the system does the only thing it knows how to do or is used to doing, and that is to take another inhale.
6. But because the lungs are partially still filled with carbon dioxide, there is less room for the fresh oxygen.
7. And the cycle continues in this line of thinking, until you stop exaggerating the inhale and figure out how to get a longer exhale.

8. That said, I am aware that there are some styles of breathing that involve exaggerated inhales that induce different states of consciousness or body awareness. This is usually done for a limited time to break down barriers and allow deep memories to surface.

EX – Breath: Exhale 2

1. As you exhale, notice where you would habitually exhale.
2. Do not consciously force or extend your exhale. Instead, notice where you would stop your exhale and don't stop it.
3. Allow your exhale to arrive at its endless destination.
4. Don't stop it…is the key phrase. There are two ways of stopping. I will explain it with walking, as it is very clear with this example.
5. Walk…stop…constrict your muscles to stop your walk.
6. Walk…stop…just stop walking. No need to overly constrict anything.
7. Try the idea of 5 and 6 with your exhale. Don't stop your exhale with constriction. Take it to its logical conclusion. Breath is your constant companion, soft and ever present. When you meet hard edges of constriction, you are up against your own resistance. When you do not limit your exhale, the tissues have the possibility of elasticity.
8. Your whole torso wants to respond to the shape changes of your exhale, informing you of your every possibility—outside, inside, thought, feeling, idea, dream state, wish, emotion. As you are reconnecting back to self, the self you left might not be the self you come back to, or the familiar self you want to come back to.

In other words, you may not want to come back to your adaptive self.

EX – Silent La La La

1. Extend your exhale without efforting.
2. Move your mouth to shape *La La La* on your exhale. But with no sound.
3. This movement tricks the glottis into staying open longer to extend your exhale.
4. Breathing is like a waterwheel, continuous. You are at the beginning, middle, or end of your inhale or exhale, the endless motion of the diaphragm.

EX – Belly Breathing

I recently watched a YouTube video of a breathing "expert" giving some tips on breathing. He sat and put his hand on his navel. He said, "Put your hand here on your diaphragm. And breathe into here, pushing your diaphragm out." I don't think he could be any more wrong.

Such misinformation. Anybody who knows anything about the diaphragm and the respiratory system knows that the diaphragm is not in your belly. As a matter of fact, the diaphragm does not ever extend below your ribcage. Never! Not possible. It attaches to the bottom of your ribcage and only rises UP from there. It never goes down to your belly. Yet this breathing expert with millions of followers was telling people it was in their belly. It is true that your belly wants to be free enough to respond to your diaphragm moving, but that is a very different process.

"Breathe into your belly" is a common directive taught in both the Yoga and Wellbeing world, as well as the Music world. But in truth if you could take the phrase literally, you would die. Breath does not go directly into your belly. Air goes into your lungs, and your belly moves to make room for it. Focusing on the abdomen triggers a downward collapse of the upper body, which creates a constriction in the chest, instead of an expansion that would make more room for air, increasing the volume of lung capacity. "Breathing into your belly" also causes a distension or doming of the abdominal wall, which creates undue pressure on the pelvic floor muscles. For women, this can negatively affect existing prolapse of the uterus and bladder.

A clarinet player I worked with told me she went to a special workshop with a top clarinet teacher, and he told her to breathe into her belly. She then came to me and told me she had so much trouble getting enough air. I told her to stop breathing into her belly, and she got the air she needed to play.

The bulk of lung tissue is in your back. If you want to direct your breath anywhere, direct it to your back, like in the next EX.

EX – Middle Back Breathing

1. Many people over-arch their back and compress the back lower spine and ribs. This interferes with the movement of the diaphragm for breathing.
2. We know the bulk of lung tissue is in your back, so you want less constriction or holding there.
3. Feel your lower ribs in your back. Then allow them to smile. A smile across your mid-back opens that area to receive more breath.

The diaphragm is like a trampoline. If one side is contracted and lacks elasticity, there is no bounce. When you can expand your lower ribs all the way around including your back, the trampoline can expand outward, then rebound in so that it bounces and the central tendon pops up. That movement activates the diaphragm chain, the dome-shaped tissues, above and below the respiratory diaphragm. The thoracic inlet and tentorium, above, and the pelvic floor and foot, below.

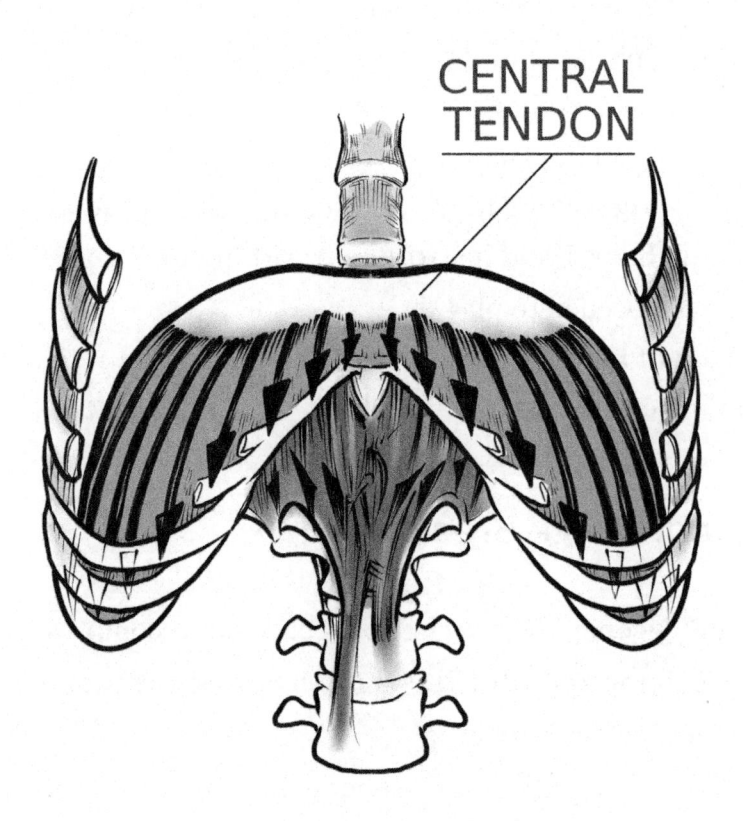

Central Tendon

II – BREATHING EXPLORACISES

EX – Element Breathing

1. Water breath – Think about water as you breathe, or a fish swimming in water. Maybe rapids on a river. Notice waves or rhythms.
2. Earth breath – Think about Earth as you breathe. Feel the solidity, stability, the rock, the support.
3. Air breath – Think about the air as you breathe, the wind that blows or the still air of summer. Air is so light and almost not there.
4. Metal breath – Think about metal as you breathe: sharp, dense, cold, solid breaths, perhaps to give you power when you need it.
5. Fire breath – Think about fire as you breathe. Feel the intensity, the inner flames that burn away what is no longer needed, or the fire of desiring something new in life.
6. First time through, think of each element.
7. Repeat and feel each element.
8. Repeat and sense each element.

EX – 5/5 Breath

I do not like to prescribe timing of breath for people, but it is interesting that many studies find that around five or six respirations per minute is healthy. That is close to breathing in for five seconds and out for five seconds. This endogenous circulatory rhythm of healthy animals and humans matches up with reciting religious prayers, like the Ave Maria, and yoga mantras. This innate rhythm modulates rhythmic fluctuations in blood pressure and heart rate as a result of autonomic control systems that are influenced by respiration, arousal, and activity. The respiratory rate (five/min) has generally favorable effects on oxygenation of the blood, and exercise tolerance. But your emotions will not let you forget that they sometimes have another tempo in mind. In other words, the 5/5 may be healthy for you, but your emotional state has another rhythm set up. Try the five in and five out and see how it is for you.

EX – The Wild Ride of Breath

1. Allow your inhale to just keep expanding by letting your ribs release. Do not force, push, or pull the inhale. It will expand on its own, seemingly, as you release your ribs. Remember that your chest opening creates a vacuum that allows the air to be pulled in.
2. When you can go no farther, let the exhale begin. Let a little air out, then stop it. Repeat many times. So your exhale has these little catches that bounce. They bounce in and then spring out to expand.
3. Eventually, these "catches" start to bounce on their own without the control of stopping the exhale. Let them. You can begin to feel this bounce of your exhale in your whole torso.
4. The bounce will stop when your exhale is complete. Wait for a moment here and feel a very deep release vibrating in your whole physicality before you begin to allow your next inhale.

EX – Lying Down Breathing

1. Lie down on your back with knees bent and feet flat.
2. Feel the energy in your feet connected to your lower back and breath.
3. Lift your ankles up a few inches and then let them down a few times. Find your rhythm.
4. Put your hands on your belly.
5. Push slightly in on your belly on your exhale.
6. Lift your ankles as you breathe in.
7. Drop your ankles and heels as you breathe out and push your belly in toward your lower back. Let your lower back lengthen. And be careful not to pull your shoulders forward. Let them stay wide.

EX – Infinity Breath with Sound

When your breath and sound fall onto your natural frequency of vibration, it feels like they can go on forever. The sound rides the breath. A natural-frequency sound is a fundamental pitch with a maximum number of overtones, and is the by-product of coordinated breathing. This sound is the key to the redevelopment of the diaphragm, as the voice is more open and resonant.

A natural-frequency sound resonates all the cells of the body, helping to keep the body healthy.

I first noticed this 30 years ago, when I was working with my teacher and mentor, breathing pioneer Carl Stough.[1] I found the concept fascinating. Vocalized breath could go on forever. When frequency, vibration, metabolic needs, and systems all coordinate and work together, we have the coherence we talked about in Chapter 2. Experiential and anatomical facts combined with emotional observations and patterns can lead to health, and to nourishing or enlightening expanded, spiritual states. Exploring deeper realms of consciousness must be done with care.

1. Exhale and begin with a few Silent La La Las.
2. On your next exhale, sound the vowel: AH as in amazing.
3. Then try these vowels: EH as in elegant.
4. EE as in eel.
5. OO as in open.
6. UU as in you.

Let each vowel go to its logical or natural conclusion, no forcing or pushing or pulling. The ancient chant of the Cathar people had AH, EH, EE, OO, UU as a recurring chorus. The Cathars were a group of people in 11th-century southern France who followed an ascetic, humanitarian way of life. They were destroyed because they threatened the religious beliefs of the times.

EX – Unity Breath

We all breathe. We have that in common. Bring your attention to your breath. Be careful. Do not force an inhale or an exhale. Notice how we tend to force. There is enough of that around. Let's allow. Pay attention instead to the easy movement of breath and the shape changes. This brings the potential to be less stuck, more able to move. Notice movement, sensation, and rhythm. As there is less constriction, the physical body and the mind settle a bit—less racing, less worry in this moment, and less habitual thinking.

As you continue watching your breath, you can sense more of your whole elastic fascial system expanding your being, connected and spacious. You can become more aware of spirit, or a larger presence. So much is unseen. Something else is present, receiving flow, and flowing in the divine. Body, mind, spirit—the unity breath. With that you can feel a bit more in yourself, with yourself, and ready to move into the world in whatever way feels right to you. Yes, the world is changing. Breath will carry you forward. Including movement, consciousness, and a connection to the world around you and something greater. Myself and the environment, near and far. Heaven, Earth, and Me… breathing together. Everyone is invited.

EX – Breathless

As I watch some modern breathing teachers, it seems to me that they are efforting so much to breathe. Forced counting and forced breath-holding is one possible style.

1. I decided to try the opposite, using as little effort as possible to breathe.
2. Basically, "can you do less" as you breathe?
3. As I used less effort, things fell away. I didn't have to draw in any air at all. I let gravity and atmospheric pressure take it in. I felt breath moving into my top nostrils and into the back of my throat.
4. Shape changes in that area seem to make a chemical change. Perhaps it is nitric oxide or the hormones from the pituitary gland.
5. At one point I think I felt the phrenic nerve spark by itself.

6. Then the most amazing thing happened. As I used less and less effort, my breathing stopped. A breath hold came on its own. Not because I forced it. I just did not need to breathe. It did not produce anxiety. It was very beautiful and very elevating.
7. A few moments later, as I continued to breathe easily and observe, I was in such a different state that I felt like I was watching myself sleep from inside. My breathing was so smooth and even. My breath was so fine. Takes my breath away.

CHAPTER 6

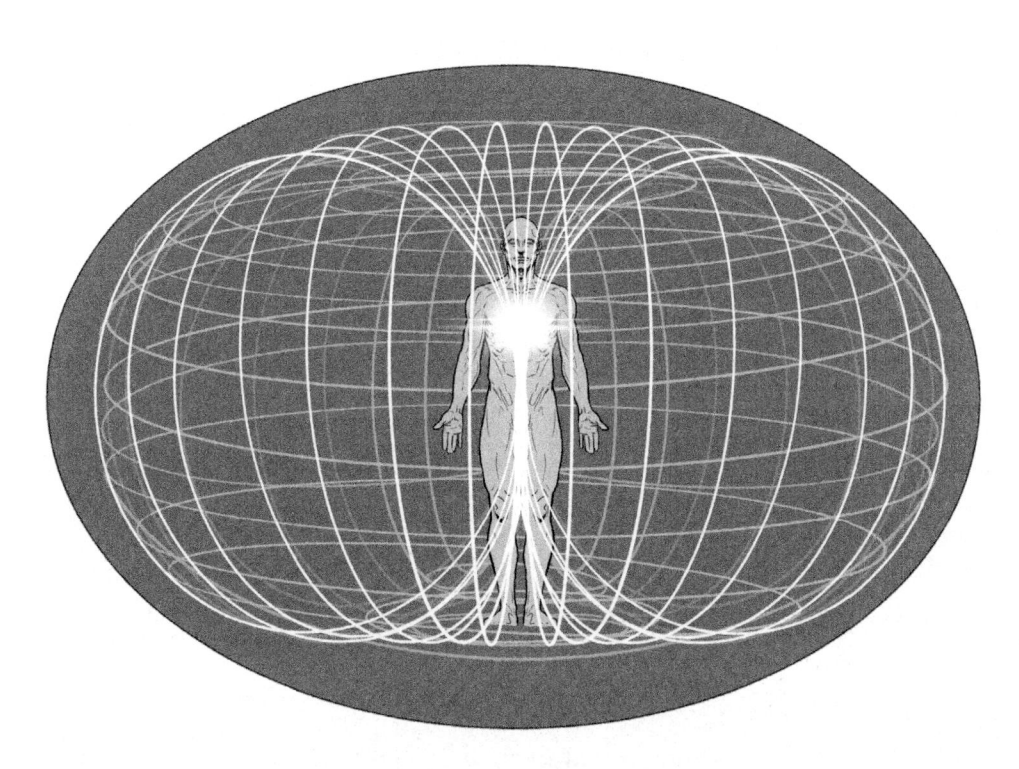

HEART

I – INTRODUCTION TO THE HEART

EX – Heart – Beginning

The heart starts to develop on day 16 after conception. Not much else has formed: no cortex, face, hands, or feet. At this time, there is a connection to Mother, including relational sensory memories, like the vibrational sound of her voice. These sensations are part of the implicit memory formed. Years ago, I saw a film that showed an embryo forming. Picture this for yourself.

1. In the early embryonic stages, your head area is rolled forward onto your chest, touching your chest.
2. With this contact the beating heart forms your face.
3. Each beat makes an indent in the face area. Amazing.
4. Maybe we are all meant to see and hear each other, and take in the world, from the beating of our hearts.

I – INTRODUCTION TO THE HEART

EX – Heart – Ending

As I mentioned earlier, according to ancient Egyptian spirituality, when you die, your heart is weighed on a scale. Let's take it into an EX. One side of the scale has your heart, and the other side has a feather of Maat (Goddess of Truth and Justice). If your heart is heavier than the feather, you need to come back to earthly life and sort out what makes your heart heavy. How would you do?

1. Sense into your own heart.
2. If you can, feel it beat.
3. Is your heart heavy?
4. Or light as a feather?

The Heart Is Not a Pump

Another medical myth tells us that the heart is a pump. It is not a pump. The idea of the pump is related to classifying the body as a machine, which it is not, as I explained in Chapter 1. Recent research suggests that the heart is a "blood spinner," a mass of tissue that folds in on itself to create a low-pressure zone within its separate chambers when emptied. The contraction of the heart-muscle tissues spins the blood into a laminated vortex as it is ejected from the ventricles, allowing the blood to move out to circulate and then to fill the heart back up. The spiraling activity catalyzes the blood to its maximum carrying capacity. The velocity and strength of the spiral motion reflect the health of the heart.[1]

As we begin to move away from the idea that the heart is simply a mechanical pump, we learn that the heart has its own nervous system that makes and releases its own neurotransmitters, and it emits an electromagnetic field that is far stronger than the brain's. The HeartMath Institute, a research and educational group in California, informs us:

> The magnetic fields produced by the heart are involved in energetic communication. The heart is the most powerful source of electromagnetic energy in the human body, producing the largest rhythmic electromagnetic field of any of the body's organs. The heart's electrical field is about 60 times greater in amplitude than the electrical activity generated by the brain. This field, measured in the form of an electrocardiogram (ECG), can be detected anywhere on the surface of the body. Furthermore, the magnetic field produced by the heart is more than 100 times greater in strength than the field generated by the brain and can be detected up to 3 feet away from the body, in all directions, using SQUID-based magnetometers.[2]

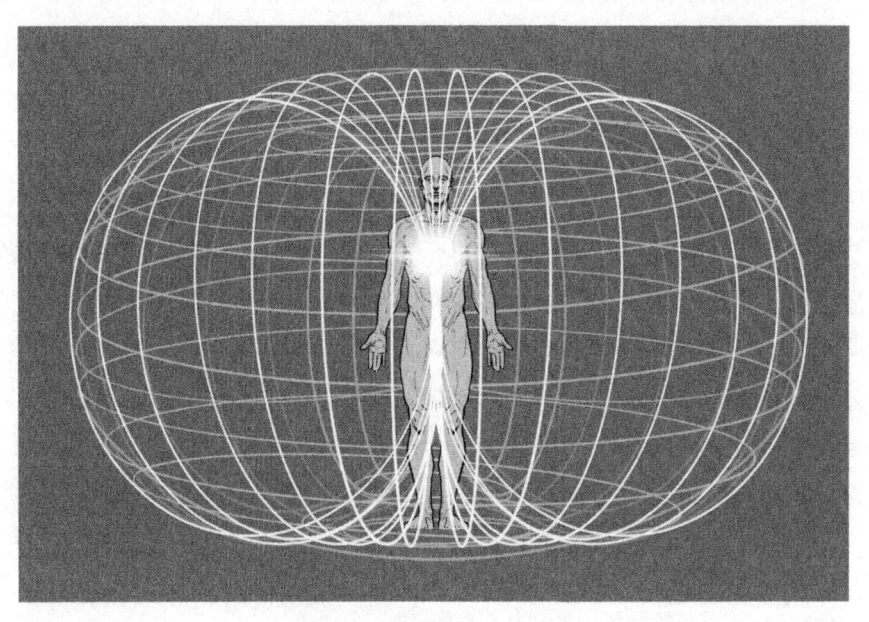

Magnetic field of the heart

1 – INTRODUCTION TO THE HEART

The heart not only has an effect on the external field surrounding the body—it has a significant influence on the internal body down to the cellular level, as the brain's rhythms along with the respiratory and blood pressure rhythms entrain with the heart's rhythm. Charles Darwin recognized the connection between heart and brain in 1872. He wrote:

> When the heart is affected, it reacts on the brain, and the state of the brain again reacts through the pneumogastric [vagus] nerve on the heart; so that under any excitement there will be much mutual action and reaction between these, the two most important organs of the body.[3]

Amazing that he knew about this coherence back then, without the sophisticated instruments we have today.

False Heart Story

Henry was having trouble with his voice. He felt wounded in his throat and heart. We started with his throat. I asked him what the wound looked like. He said it was heart-shaped. He felt a heart in his throat that interfered with his voice. With that, he said it was like he crawled into a deep hole, a place to heal, surrounded by dirt. It was pleasant. He felt the wound was a little soothed, but there seemed to be more healing to do.

Since the wound was in front, I had him pay attention to his back to balance it, the back of his head, his sacrum, and his heels. His voice became clearer as he did this. He remembered that his father had a job that he was concerned about and often talked to Henry about it, but Henry did not want to talk about his father's job. He was looking for holding, nurturing, and love from his father. Henry had pain in his heart. Because of the pain in his heart, he had to close down his heart, and then his system created a small heart in his throat. A false heart. The false heart does not function well in his throat, so it became a problem for his voice. We often think of the adaptive pattern as behavioral. But in this case, it became structural. The false heart was protection, armor. Back to Wilhelm Reich, the father of somatic therapy, and creator of the term *armoring.* All somatic roads lead to Reich. Henry started to move his neck very gently. The muscles in the neck have five bony attachments: to skull, spine, upper arm, jaw, and ribs. Each of these attachments seemed to release as Henry moved his neck, processed the emotion, and allowed his breath to settle. As he opened his eyes and his awareness came back to the room, the muscles around his eyes relaxed. There was a ventral connection with a clearer voice, and more social connection. The false heart that Henry had developed was no longer necessary, and he was able to drop down and settle in his true heart.

II – HEART EXPLORACISES

Given its diverse fields of influence, the word "heart" is used in many different contexts: the heart of humanity; the heart of the matter; home is where the heart is; heart-centered; change of heart; cross my heart; heart of gold; cry your heart out; eat your heart out; have a heart; follow your heart; total eclipse of the heart; broken heart; heart of stone; young at heart; my heart goes out to you; sacred heart, to name a few.

EX – Physicality of the Heart of Humanity

During a crisis (such as the pandemic), we see that people reach out more than usual. Somehow our perceptions change, and our hearts are able to be touched. How and when does that opening happen? Perhaps our answer lies in thinking/feeling more along the lines of less judgment or blame, and more compassion or understanding.

1. Let's look at the physicality of blaming from a fearful state. What position does your body take when you are blaming someone?
2. Often, there is a kind of tightness in the front of the face and heart, as the finger points to blame.
3. In contrast, let's look at the physicality of understanding or compassion from a loving state.
4. Often, there is a softening and opening of the heart, as if to let the other person's point of view in. It is often said that the longest journey is from head to heart.
5. When we become aware of heart qualities, they have an impact on our health, wellbeing, and connection to those around us. As we move into the Aquarian Age of increased peace, harmony, love, and concern for the whole human race, we become more heart-centered, and less fearful. Love is the opposite of fear. Astrological ages shift around every 2,000 or so years, and each age has different influences.

EX – A Lakota Teaching

1. There is a door in the heart that lets evil spirits in. All prayer is strengthening your heart to guard this door. So, fear stays outside the door and does not come into your heart.
2. Practicing this would help our world.

II – HEART EXPLORACISES

EX – Broken Heart

Early experiences of hurt or neglect can cause the heart to close, and the chest to collapse. The heart does not want to open again, as a return of the pain would be too great to bear. Providing support for the heart can ease this pain. The physical placement of your heart offers an immediate picture of support.

1. The heart sits on top of your diaphragm.
2. Every time you breathe in or out, your heart moves.
3. As you exhale, your diaphragm domes up inside your ribcage to support and hold your heart from the bottom. This is another good reason to extend your exhale when possible.
4. It is almost like your heart gets an internal massage from your breath.
5. On your back, the surface layer of muscles gathers between your shoulder blades and supports your heart from the back. This is not pulling your shoulder blades together as in "good posture," but rather a gentle gathering to hold your heart.
6. The heart, diaphragm, and pericardium all wrapped up together can be a wonderful inner resource when your heart feels broken, for personal or global reasons.

EXPLORACISES

EX – Heart–Pelvis Disconnect

As I have been doing hands-on work for many years, I notice that many people have a lot of holding and tightness in their upper body. Energetically, there is stiff energy held in the upper torso and very little energy in the lower torso. This can be seen visually and sensed energetically. This disconnect between upper and lower torso sometimes means that the heart is not involved in the pelvic decisions. This may be fun for a while, but one can quickly lose interest and go on to look for the next person to satisfy one's needs. Yet it may never be truly satisfying if the heart is not involved.

1. Become aware of the tightness in your upper body. This will manifest in held breath, lack of motility in the ribs, and/or tight shoulders.
2. Place one hand on the top of your sternum, below your collarbones. Stay there for a few breaths and see if you can feel the movement of your breath.
3. Begin to gently encourage your sternum to release and soften.
4. Direct your sternum and the breath's movement down toward your toes. And down toward your spine.
5. See if you can begin to let the energy travel down to your lower torso. As the energy in your torso evens out and becomes more balanced, you may feel tingling in your whole torso.
6. You may feel a little emotional as your heart releases.
7. What does it feel like to have your heart and pelvis connected?

II – HEART EXPLORACISES

EX – Moving into Life with the Heart Leading the Way

1. Bring your attention to your feet, where there is often a bracing pattern. The foot complex contains 26 bones, 33 joints, and more than 100 muscles, tendons, and ligaments. Considering both feet, that is a total of 52 bones, making up about a quarter of all bones found in the mature adult body.
2. Explore micro-movements, the tiny movements in your feet, moving all 52 bones.
3. Rest your feet.
4. Bring your attention to your heart. Put your right hand on your left ribs near your heart. Put your left hand on your right upper arm. This is a heart hug. Holding. Maybe you want someone else to hold you. But now you hold yourself. Feel what that feels like inside you.
5. Heaven can be accessed through the pineal gland in the head, the sixth chakra. Earth is accessed through the base of the torso, the root chakra. They meet in the middle in the heart. Any decision made by the mind will have polarity, two sides to it. Only decisions made by the heart can be in the unified field, with oneness for all.[4]
6. As you hug the deep heart that emerges when Heaven and Earth meet in synchronized embodiment, how is that for you? There is a lot of suffering on the planet now. Some of it is hard to take in. There is also a growing strong hope that we as a collective will make choices that will sustain life and our planet.
7. Go back to your feet and feel the heart hug and feet together.

8. You feel the inner movement of your feet and then picture the outer movement, as if your feet are moving you forward in life.
9. Get up and walk. Think of your feet moving you into the life you want, led by your deep heart and the wonderful unifying electromagnetic energy it gives out.

EX – Origins of the Pattern and Heartbeat

1. Name one of your physical, tensing, constrictive patterns.
2. Name the place it shows up in your body.
3. Where is the spot it seems to initiate from?
4. Where is the engine that starts this seemingly necessary and driven pattern?
5. Observe what small micro-movements might be happening there, such as pulsing or pulling—the movements that are already there giving the pattern its life support.
6. You visit the pattern where it is. Do not bring it to you. Watch it move.
7. Is there an emotion or perception there? Perhaps profound desperation, sadness, terror, disconnection, or longing?
8. Do you have the ability to see how everything you do, say, think, feel, sense, is based on this initial pattern? Often, we are aware of the pattern but don't seem to be able to touch or change it.

For me now as I ask these questions, I hear and feel my heartbeat. I recognize that the rest of me must be very quiet for me to feel and hear my heartbeat. There seems to be some information here for me. I feel my heartbeat reverberating out through the rest of me, in synchronized embodiment. This seems to be the only way possible to touch the pattern, though I just said that it seems impossible to change. But with the love I feel, there is so much more responsibility somehow to include the whole fascial network, all of me. As great mystical spiritual teachers have taught over the years, the path forward is love. But that is not always easy to believe. Today as I feel my heartbeat reverberate through my being, when I can quiet the rest of me, then the love becomes real for me. I was not breathing to the heart, but allowing the heart to breathe, as in the illustration in the introduction of this book.

Not something that somebody taught me but a true blessing, gift, miracle from inside. Finding the initiation to my matrix, pattern, puzzle. Finding the micro-movements there, and the emotion there. And I once thought the pattern could never change, because the pattern was built to survive. Finding my heartbeat. The vibration of my heartbeat was the only possible way to touch the foundational pattern of survival. I am now at rest. Resting in my own breath. I wrote this on Easter. Happy Easter—death and rebirth.

CHAPTER 7

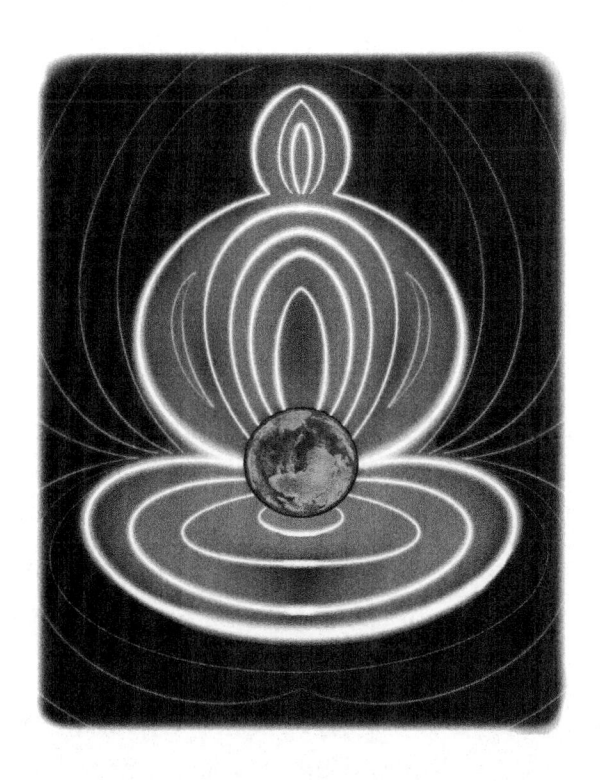

SPIRIT AND MEDITATION

I – INTRODUCTION TO SPIRITUALITY

The planet and humanity are facing multiple challenges impacting both individuals and the collective. Many are obvious. But the greatest danger is less obvious. The greatest danger we face is the internal loss of consciousness in daily life, not any external situation. Our spirituality lives in this consciousness. Yet many live at the mercy of unconscious patterns of fear, anger, and lack of empathy. The choice for our evolutionary journey seems to be between unconscious egoic *me, me,* or a more awakened consciousness of *we is the new me*, as we also maintain individual sovereignty. Then perhaps we will not lose consciousness in daily life and end up as a barcode. Let's make the right choices…

I – INTRODUCTION TO SPIRITUALITY

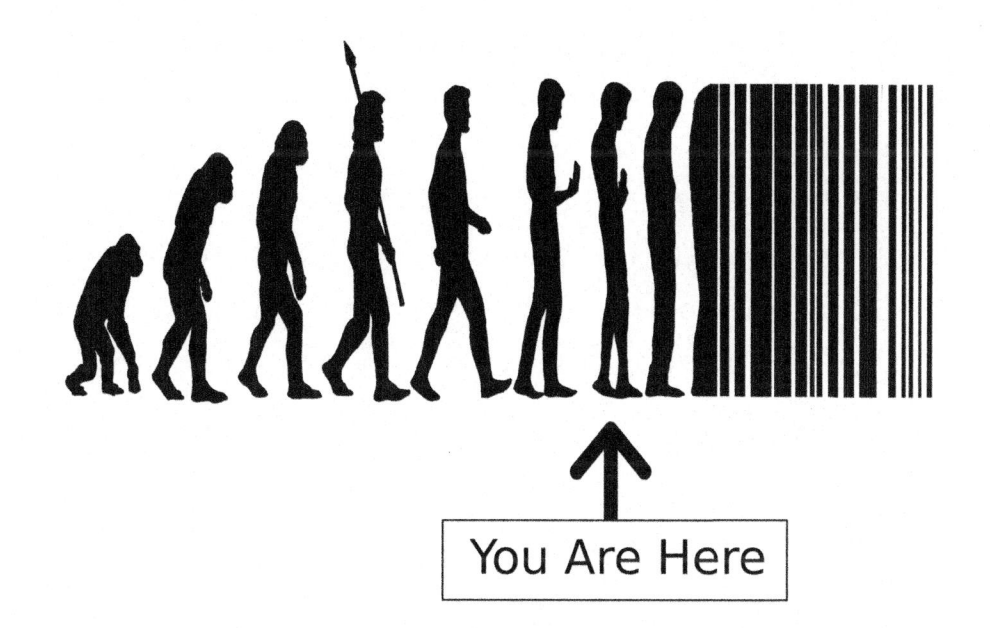

Choice

EX – What If It Wasn't This?

It is said that in the Bible the word "stiff-necked" appears more than 300 times.[1] Its implied meaning is that we have rigid, stubborn, fixed ideas.

1. Pay attention to your head. Any physical holding or psychological stuck thoughts?
2. Pay attention to your shoulders. Any physical holding or psychological stuck thoughts? The psychology is in your tissues, membranes, and fibers.
3. Pay attention to what is in between your head and shoulders: your neck, a passageway with many forms and functions,

including breath, voice, spine, nervous system. Any physical holding or psychological stuck thoughts, replaying tapes?

4. Is any of this stiff-necked? Do you have rigid thoughts and beliefs?
5. Think of something that you think is true.
6. What if it wasn't true? What if it wasn't this? Stay with this idea.
7. Can you have some sense of less stiffness in your neck that might allow your beliefs and fixed ideas to change, and to include some other possibilities?

EX – Words to Meditate On

- White light speaking: "I am just a beam of light traveling on this planet. Darkness touches me sometimes."
- Organic divinity exists.
- Some doors open only from the inside, like breath.
- Thinking can be a disease.
- Biology is a printout of the mind.
- Ego expansion vs. universal expansion.
- The Red Sea parted—when water was at the heads of the people during the Exodus in the Hebrew Bible.
- Step and the floor will appear. The floor appears after you step, not before.
- Be seen by someone who is not you.
- What is it in life that you cannot do?
- Everything comes from the silence.
- Guilt is *I am bad and full of ego.* Regret is *I wish I had known better.*

I – INTRODUCTION TO SPIRITUALITY

EX – The Pineal Gland

The pineal gland is our "third eye" and the organ through which we dream and imagine. It is also the organ that connects us to other dimensions of reality, such as time travel, astral journeying, or the development of psychic skills (clairvoyance or telepathy, for example). Many religions claim to have a monopoly on connecting us with divinity, but actually, the temple to reach divine connection is within each of us.

Although medically not proven, it is said that in some circumstances, the pineal gland can produce a substance called DMT (dimethyltryptamine), also known as "the spiritual molecule," that is responsible for visualizing images in dreams. The powerful DMT can carry our consciousness through time travel and dimensions. It can achieve mystical states and has profound effects on consciousness. Meditation offers an opening to practice and grow our connection to our pineal gland, the mind-body-spirit temple of the divinity within us.

1. The pea-sized pineal gland is in the middle of your brain in a groove just above the thalamus.
2. From the crown of your head, make a plumbline down.
3. The pineal gland is above your ears.
4. Meditate on your pineal gland.

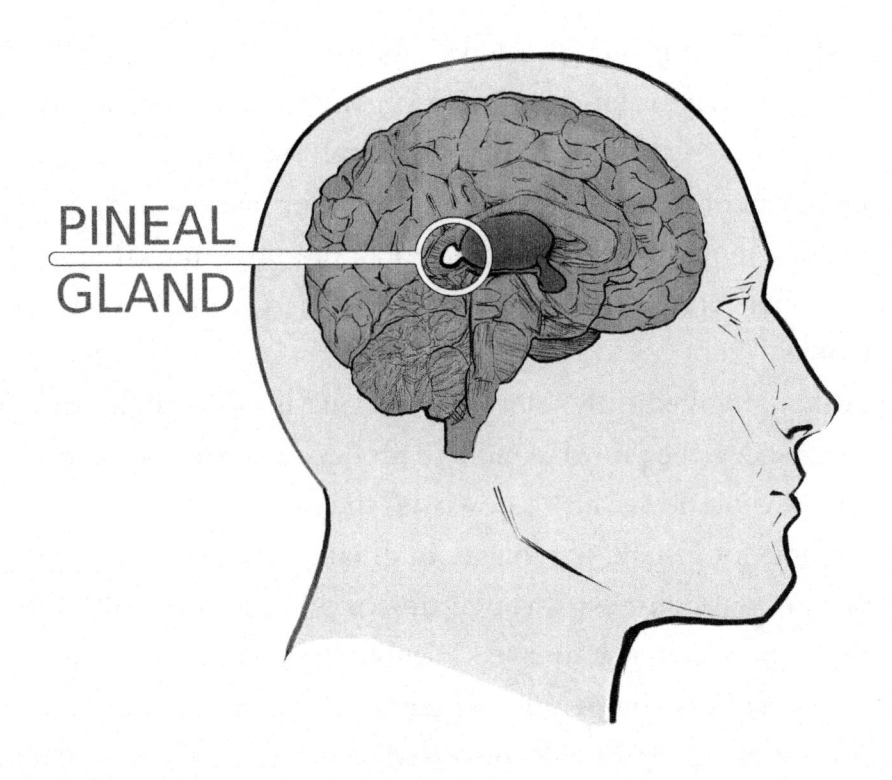

Pineal Gland

II – MEDITATION EXPLORACISES

EX – Meditation Recalibration

We need both spirit and emotion, Heaven and Earth.

1. You start to meditate.
2. Perhaps you see white light and beautiful images. You would like to just dwell there.
3. But something inside gnaws at you. It is the knots and tangling in your belly that are part of your bracing pattern.
4. Bring the light to your belly, belly central. Hold both, the beautiful light and the tangled belly.
5. Breath changes. Some movement happens. Recalibration is going on.
6. Part of you wants to return to just spirit, so inviting, so tempting. But if you do that, the next moment you get upset, your peace will all fly out the window.

7. You must take care of the upset twisting and contractions. This is the only way out, to real freedom—holding the upset with the beautiful white light that so graciously appears to you.

This is not an exercise. It is an *EXploracise,* done with excruciating awareness of the bracing patterns and strong pulls. No need, for now, to know why they exist. Your belly contractions quiver, shake, and tremble, like the tectonic plates of the Earth, like so many earthquakes now. So much held trauma that is not addressed. The bracing patterns are so strong, no amount of surface exercise will help foundationally. You need to cultivate inner attention.

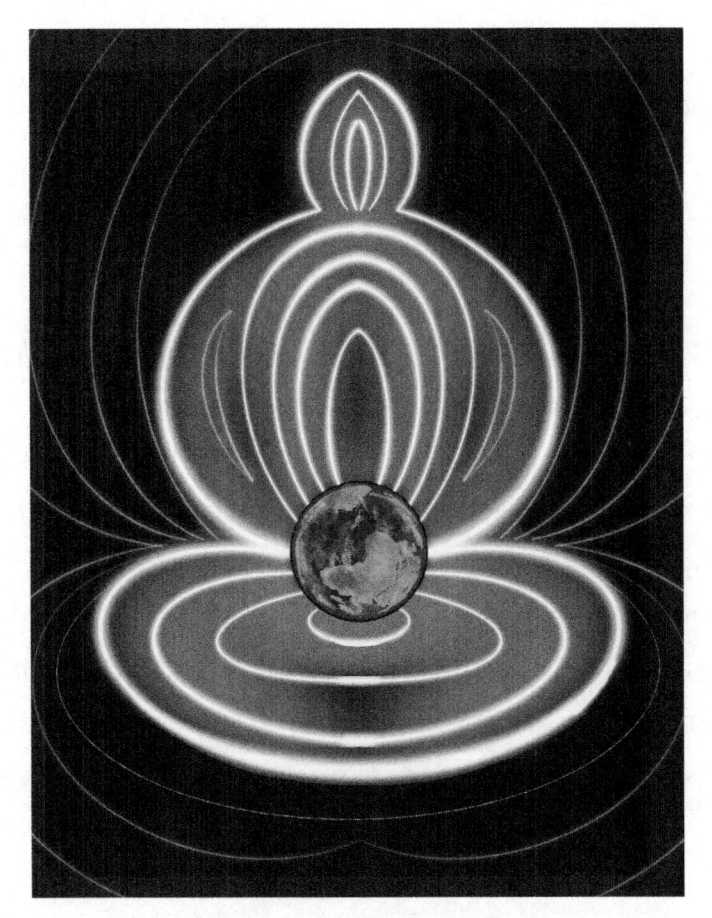

Buddha Meditation

II – MEDITATION EXPLORACISES

EX – Meditation: Is the State You Want the State You Are In?

1. See where you are. What is going on in your bodily reactions and responses? Any thinking, racing, moving, or repeating? What emotion is there? Recognize that we are motivated by emotion all the time.
2. What changes happen as you become aware of all this?
3. Is the state you want the state you are in? Or is it a state you are not thrilled about? You may want to be loving and content, but you actually feel angry or anxious.
4. What do we do with that? Anger or fear is not what I want to be feeling, but it IS what I'm feeling.
5. Recognize where you are. And recognize your support and contact with the ground that is under you.
6. As that happens, there is a chance of softening or an invitation for breath.
7. As you watch breath, some movement can occur: your torso, chest, or belly has potential movement.
8. As your chest moves, your heart is touched. Do you have compassion for yourself and what is happening? Recognizing that you do not have compassion is a practice that can lead you to having compassion.
9. The movement of your heart affects the whole of you: physical, mental, emotional, and spiritual, your life force.
10. Stay with that a moment, and recognize the possibility of your state changing, so that the state you are in is the state you want.

EXPLORACISES

Variation: EX – Background Noise Contemplation

1. Take a minute to see where you are.
2. Observe what is happening in your outer environment. Then recognize what is happening in your inner environment.
3. Do they match?
4. Is there any background activity going on inside that doesn't match the outer environment? Perhaps you are sitting in a beautiful field of flowers, but you feel the jitteriness of anxiety inside as a background.
5. Is what is happening inside you an appropriate response to what is happening outside you? Are they congruent? Often there is a background noise inside that doesn't really match the immediate environment.
6. If that is true, see what happens when you recognize that.
7. What happens if you pay attention to the background noise inside? What happens to your breathing? What happens to your ability to be aware of your support? Does awareness allow that to shift or downregulate?
8. When you look around again, do you see your environment differently?

II – MEDITATION EXPLORACISES

EX – Shape-Changes Meditation: Your Body Is the Printout

Meditation where you observe your thoughts is one style, and meditation where you notice emerging somatic messages is another.

1. What are the voices in your head telling you this morning?
2. How does your body manifest that? What does it look, feel, sense like? Your body is the printout of your mind, emotion, and invisible being. (Think of the modern 3D printer that can create tools or furniture.)
3. There are possible shape changes. They touch your breathing, the delicacy of breath, the soft edges of breath.
4. Notice the changes of shape inside your body. As your body moves, the changes affect the air around you, and everything around you.
5. How willing and able is your system to shift, change, adjust, and move to meet changing circumstances? These days there are many.
6. Recognize the contact with the ground and what is under you. How does that affect those small changes?

These small changes are often skipped over, and yet the nervous and fascial systems are well-attuned to observe and absorb small changes. Being able to be aware of these small changes is a first step. Then listen to them. As you train yourself to listen to small shifts and go with them, you are better able to handle the big shifts as they come. The idea that "I can change" can be helpful when times are difficult and we are forced to change. Can we go with it?

EX – Tongue on the Roof of Your Mouth

1. Allow as much of your tongue as possible to rest on the roof of your mouth.
2. At the same time it is resting on the roof of your mouth, if possible, have your tongue make contact with the soft palate, which is at the back of your mouth. (You can feel it with your finger.)
3. The soft palate energetically meets the top of your spine, creating an electric charge.
4. As you meditate here, electric energy spreads to your whole body.

EX – Crown Chakra Meditation

The top of your head is called your *crown chakra,* and it is one of your main subtle-energy centers.

1. Allow the energy from the Heavens, above your head, to enter your body through this center.
2. As this enters your body, you can allow it to travel down.
3. Either to your heart.
4. Or travel right down through you to meet the Earth energy that is coming up.
5. You can think of the two energies meeting and moving in a spiral shape.

II – MEDITATION EXPLORACISES

EX – Meeting Points of Balance to Come Together

1. Allow your weight to shift side to side as you sit. Feel the weight changes. Where are you heavy or light?
2. How is breath on each side?
3. As you go from side to side, you pass through the center. That center point is the middle of an X, where your two sides meet, your center.
4. We can expand this to the outer world.
5. The center in myself, my own X, meets the X in you, and there is an X meeting point between us. We become one.
6. Expand it out and many around the globe can become one in that moment. In trauma, personal or the collective, things get fragmented and come apart. In this moment we find the meeting point of coming together in ourselves and each other.
7. We can all meditate on coming together.

EX – Sides Meditation

1. As you breathe, allow your side ribs to move.
2. Let your diaphragm tuck up under your side ribs, so your side ribs drape downward on your exhale.
3. Your side ribs relate to the corners of your mouth, and to your two sides of your underarms, and to your two hip crests.
4. Meditate on the relationships of the horizontal nature of these sides.
5. The strong sense of letting go downward is not due to dropping your shoulders—it is your ribs that you want to drop down.

As the sides of your ribs drop down, you feel the joints in your sternum release to allow this or vice versa. But either way, your ribs letting go downward allows you to feel relief in your whole body. Maybe with a sigh.

6. Your shoulders want to stay mobile and go along for the ride. Do not hold or pull your shoulders down.
7. Any stuck place in your sternum can be a bit less stuck. Your sternum floats. As the sides of the ribs go down, the sternum goes up, allowing your shoulders to release.

EX – Meditation and Breath

Used in many styles of yoga, *ujjayi pranayama* is a breathing technique that produces an ocean-like sound. It involves inhaling through the nose and exhaling through the mouth while constricting the throat to create a "ha" sound. Forced "ujjayi breath" may be good for changing your state of consciousness, but not good for your throat if you do it by tightening your pharynx as much as possible, especially if you have any kind of voice trauma. I think it is possible to produce a type of *ujjayi* without the strong constriction. I seem to have stumbled upon it.

1. One day, I was meditating watching breath go in and out.
2. All of a sudden, there was this deep vibratory sound in my throat that seemed to come from engaging or enlivening the muscles there.
3. Something deep in the back of my throat seemed to be affected.

4. I was not doing something to make it happen. It came from an openness, and not from a closing. This is a big difference! Explore this possibility.

Many techniques try to imitate a natural process that arises from non-doing or sensing. They try to imitate it with a forced, ego-driven, alpha duplication that seems right, on the surface, but does not really have the depth of the original process.

Maybe this can be likened to an actor trying to duplicate a performance by copying the outer movement of something that worked as an inner process. If it was right in one moment, it may never be right again. It is ego: *I am doing* vs. whole self: *allowing and sensing*.

EX – Meditating with Energetic Pain

This morning in my meditation, I felt such discomfort. It was too painful to:

1. Release my shoulder blades, so they could support my heart in back.
2. Let the thoracic inlet open, and let the trigeminal, aka cranial nerve 5, connect to my body, and let my face express what my body was feeling. Cranial nerve 5 allows the face to show what the body is feeling. If the feeling is too uncomfortable, it doesn't show. Energetic pain can be emotional or physical or both.
3. I wanted to allow a pattern of healthy organization, but I could not. It was way too painful.

    Often, I talk about the child who feels pain in her body that is so overwhelming that she goes to her head to escape the pain. Well, I felt it today. It is real. My body was too painful and too chaotic to feel. I did not want to force my body back, even though I could have forced my physicality into comfort with breath or manipulation.

4. Instead, I remembered that via swinging motions like a pendulum, chaos can return to organization. So, in my body I became aware of the chaotic pattern of the pain, although it was not really chaotic; it was very familiar and patterned. But it was out of synchrony with wellbeing or ventral vagal. As I gently swung my body side to side, I watched the chaotic pattern. It slowly returned to a higher state of organization.
5. If you disturb a system a little, then support it, it can organize to a higher state.
6. I was willing to feel the disturbed physical system, the emotional dysregulation, and then to support it—and it reorganized, with the swinging, to a higher state of presence, homeostasis, and effective function.
7. I can now bear the emotional, energetic, and physical pain as it shifts or when it shifts because of my presence, and then I can bear it because it has changed.
8. An observation about the word *homeostasis*. Stasis implies it is static. But everything inside us is constantly adjusting in each moment, very far from static. Perhaps *homeodynamic* works better. In this book, I will use homeostasis, as it is the common verbiage.

II – MEDITATION EXPLORACISES

EX – My Morning Meditation

1. I focus my brain as I watch breath come in and go out. I feel my brain struggling to stay in one spot that seems to be in the middle front of my brain.
2. I add gentle, flowing movement. I watch the movement in my body but stay connected to this spot in my brain. I watch them move together.
3. I realize that I need to accept everything just as it is, painful or good. I must accept it. There seems to be no other way. If I don't accept it, what am I fighting against? When you fight with yourself, who wins? What is happening is real. What I think should happen is not real.
4. I stay with that, difficult as it may be. I feel the oneness in my whole body, mind, self. I remember the words I wrote in *HUMANUAL*.[2] The ideas of unity and expansion take on new meaning. I experience this expanded oneness deep in my psyche and bones. Expansion extends both inward and outward in our physicality.
5. There is a oneness. Call it the Divine, God, Spirit, or whatever you like. But it is real. I feel it. My brain holds it or stays with it, and my body feels and senses it. They all work together. The togetherness is the togetherness of the entire world spinning together.
6. I realize it must be love. The oneness is love. I feel it. Even though I am in grief about the world being destroyed by greedy individuals, this process cracks open a space to see the oneness and the love.

EXPLORACISES

7. I open my eyes from meditation and consciously let my brain see from this deep center. My body joins this glorious encounter with the world. I move through life. And this will be my teaching for all who want to listen.

CHAPTER 8

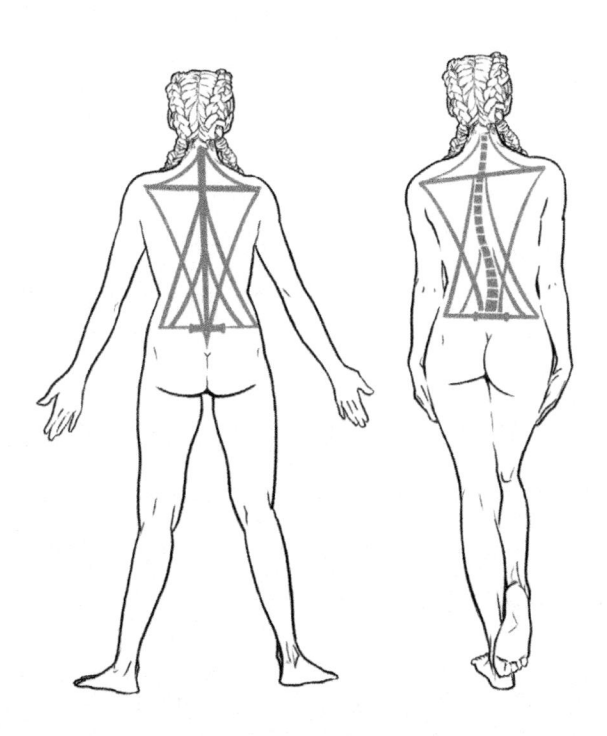

EMOTION

I – INTRODUCTION TO EMOTION

I would like to start this chapter on emotion with this touching story about Charlie Chaplin. Sir Charles Spencer Chaplin KBE, an English comic actor, filmmaker, and composer, told a funny story at one of his shows. The whole audience laughed a lot. He told the same funny story a little later in the performance, and about half the audience laughed. He told the funny story a third time in the performance, and no one laughed. He then asked the audience, "Why do you not laugh at the funny story the third time, but you cry over and over for the same sad story?" What happens inside as you read the last line?

Emotions are not random; they happen for a reason. They are also the biggest thing in the room, as they call attention to feeling states. Your physiology responds to emotions every second. They show up in your heart, belly, or just about anywhere as general pressures. Sometimes it's just a whiff of emotion; other times it feels like a ton of bricks and lasts forever. Sometimes emotion is so loud that you cannot sleep, and other times it's a faint voice that reminds you of something

I – INTRODUCTION TO EMOTION

from your past. We cannot live without our emotional connections. We want to normalize and validate them.

When we are young, we cry because we are pained with needs. We hope our mother figure or caregiver will come, as they are our emotional connection. If no one comes, the need is not met, there is no connection, and the pain is not soothed. This causes separation and distress, leading to a possibility of the danger of abandonment. Connection to others who give us food, shelter, and nurturing is our survival. We need a safe haven. If we don't get one, we continue to look with hypervigilance for the safety. Sadly, this can go on into future development, and present emotions become the end product of these past experiences.

Emotional isolation destroys us, and we call the result of that *trauma*. We need to let emotions move and not block them, as we are pliable beings, an ongoing creation that is not rigid.

II – EMOTION EXPLORACISES

EX – Welcome Baby

When your parental figures did not welcome you, it made sense to pull your arms in. You opened to the caregivers, but they were not available, so you pulled in little by little. Like falling down a staircase and crumpling, pulled in.

Now to change the pattern:

1. Close your eyes and go back to the moment you reached out to them and imagine a new, different caregiver there who would welcome you. Feel that in your arms.
2. Feel the reach out in your arms.
3. Let the reach bounce in the direction it is going until it hits a stop.
4. Then as a reaction your arms will pull back in.
5. Go back and forth between the reach out and the pull in, in tiny movements. The important part here is the connection

between the pull in and reach out. You are not just manipulating a correction to reach out. You feel each and every step of the pull in and the reach out. If you just manipulate it out, it is not the part of you that created the pattern. The you that created the pattern is the pull in. Honor the concept of "I need to pull in."

6. Notice that the movement of your arms includes your heart. As you pull your arms in, your heart retreats and constricts. As you reach your arms forward, your shoulders anchor on your back, and your heart can expand and be supported from your back.

EX – Envision or Recall Your Young Self

A horse can walk soon after it is born. A human baby does not walk until 10 or 12 months. Animals are preprogrammed. We are not. Most human connections get made in that first year. Humans are greatly influenced and formed by the environment. How could it be otherwise? That is our thinking, behaving, and bracing pattern for life—until we decide that the adaptive pattern is now maladaptive. Imagine some of your early environment.

1. Go back to your young self. Imagine: How did you move? How did you breathe?
2. Who did you talk to?
3. What did it feel like?
4. How did you hold difficult emotions inside?
5. What was your coping strategy to endure when your needs were not met?
6. What was the posture of the parent or caregiver who had no time to talk to you?

7. What was the posture of the parent who was approachable?
8. Children like to move. Do you remember the joy of movement?

EX – Your Birthday

A friend was telling me about their child's birthday party. She said she asked him if he wanted a party. How many people? What kind of cake? He went to the bakery and helped choose the cake. His emotions and feelings were involved in planning his party. At first, I thought to myself, *this is nuts.* He is going to be three years old. Then I thought more about it.

1. What if I was offered those choices for my third birthday? My little three-year-old self was shocked and could barely imagine what I might want. But I quickly began to see and feel what I did and did not want for my birthday party.
2. Go to your three-year-old self and decide how you want to spend your birthday, the celebration of your life.

EX – Conversations in Your Head

1. As you listen to the conversations in your head, let your body move with them. As we know, when you are having thoughts, your body is a printout of the thoughts.
2. See what happens when you let the expressive thoughts move fully.
3. Take up space.

II – EMOTION EXPLORACISES

4. "I told you not to do that." "Will he ever listen to me?" "They violated our agreement." "I am so happy today."
5. As you move, what is underneath—what emotion? Anger, joy, sadness? Be with that. All issues are in our tissues.

EX – Emotional Tensegrity

1. When you feel down, dejected, or depressed, mentally make a tensegrity structure. Name all the emotions on the meeting points of the structure: sad, grieving, depressed, anxious, unworthy, unloved.
2. When you feel joy, do the same with the positive emotions that you feel: happy, content, joyous, loved, welcomed, connected, safe.
3. Some days you may have a mixture.
4. As you name all the points on the tensegrity structure, note the oneness of the tensegrity and the ability to have many different aspects in that oneness.
5. If you are so inclined, you can draw your emotional tensegrity.

EX – Meditation to Balance Emotions

The Secret of the Golden Flower: A Chinese Book of Life teaches that we want to balance our emotions for true contentment. It is a practical guide to the integration of personality, and a natural way to mental freedom.[1]

1. Joy, surrender, peace, courage, will, truth, love are the emotions this book suggests emphasizing.
2. Take a moment to find balance in yourself with each one: joy, surrender, peace, courage, will, truth, love.
3. Can you balance joy, surrender, peace, courage, will, truth, love all together on your tensegrity structure?
4. Can you balance them in your family, community, and beyond?

EX – Shadow Dance

1. Become aware of your pain in one spot.
2. Feel the tightness under the pain. Feel the direction that the tightness is pulling.
3. Find the shadow of the pull and let it move around the pull. You are not moving tight muscles, but the shadow surrounding them. You are moving the fascia.
4. Explore this with your chosen spot.
5. Rest.
6. Now choose the next spot. Then the next, then the next, and the next.
7. Let the shadows of two spots knit together, and move together. Then three, then four, etc.
8. Move all the shadows of the spots off or away from the bracing pattern.

Remember, do not move individual muscles. Try to move the shadow, or surrounding area. Shadow-dance all together. Let the pattern have its movement. A change will come as indicated by breath, emotion, or a yawn. To understand the body as healer, pay attention, and the body will heal. Divine light spreads everywhere and has no shadow.[2]

EX – A Twist of Bad

1. Something in the environment is not good, so it is either it or you that is the problem.
2. If it, your survival is threatened, and it might not be able to care for you. So, in self-defense, you choose you as the part that is not good—and that makes you bad.
3. Then realizing that you are bad, you do everything in your power to convince people that you are not bad.
4. You even lose touch with your own badness. You become so skilled at trying to be good, you don't even know you have a shadow side.

EX – Catch Your Emotional Adaptive Patterns

As Sally was shopping in the grocery store, a very well-dressed, cool woman approached. Sally immediately saw herself try to look cool. Then she stopped, thinking to herself, *"What are you doing?"* There was her adaptive pattern: trying to be like someone else, because she, herself, was not okay.

Frank was having a great day, so he was dancing down the hallway in his apartment building. He saw someone approaching and stiffened up. This was his adaptive pattern: *"Don't let anyone see me really happy."*

Both examples involve:

1. Some kind of constriction to stop the natural flow.
2. Loss of communication with oneself and others, with the stiffening.
3. Perceived lack of safety to show oneself.
4. When can you catch your adaptive pattern?

EX – Changing the Lived Experience / My Movie / Fear No More

Mentally bring up a difficult incident. Explore before, during, and after it. For example: "I am going to my boss for my review."

1. Go through the movie of just the facts of what happened before, during, and after.
   I was walking toward the office. I went in. He spoke a few words. I left. Just the facts of the story.
2. Go through it now and add emotion:
   As I was walking toward the office, I felt excitement, realizing I did a good job, and I wanted him to acknowledge that. I felt joy. In the office he said I did well, and that was it. No compliments or encouragement. I experienced disappointment. As I walked out, I experienced dejection and abandonment.
3. Go through this "movie" again and feel the associated bodily sensations.
   Excitement was tingly, upbeat, and bubbly. In the office I started to feel heavy and closed in on myself. As I walked away, my sensations were frozen and constricted.

11 – EMOTION EXPLORACISES

4. Go through it, exploring your breath as it happened.
   Breath was freely moving. Then sort of constricted. Then barely breathing.
5. Go through it with movement.
   At first, I was skipping along to his office. As he spoke, I started to squirm. I was dragging my feet as I left.

Is the sequence familiar to you? Can you recall a childhood experience that is similar in emotion but not similar in facts? For example:

1. I came home from school with a good grade, excited to tell my parents (the expectation).
2. My mother was busy and barely responded. My father was working (the actual happening).
3. I went to my room feeling sad (my response).
4. *I feel alone.* The result I am left with is the imprint.
5. Go back to the adult story and go through the steps, noticing your breath.
6. And again with movement. Maybe exaggerate the movement.

The story facts are the same, but my lived experience of it is different. When we are young, we are one with our caregivers. We take on their breath, movement, and emotional blocks. As we get older and separate, we often take those with us. Then we realize—*that is not mine. I don't have or like that block. Maybe my boss was having a bad day, and his lack of enthusiasm had nothing to do with me.*

III – ANGER

Anger comes up: when you don't get what you think you deserve, or when you get what you think you don't deserve. The feeling is often immediate and strong, affecting your whole body, especially your jaw and shoulder.

Healthy anger is a boundary defense. If someone comes too close and wants to hurt you or take something from you, be it tangible or not, you want to protect yourself. Expressing anger in the moment it is happening is a healthy response.

This protective aspect is comparable to the immune system, which defends and protects against toxic substances. We let in good feelings, and we keep out harmful advances. We let in good bacteria and keep out toxic substances. A compromised emotional system often breeds a compromised immune system.

When possible, do not push anger down inside. Anger that is not expressed in the moment, for one reason or another, gets held inside and builds into rage, and feels like it may explode in any moment.

III – ANGER

After you express healthy anger, your system can recalibrate back to homeostasis.

EX – Deep Anger

1. Remember a time in your life when you wanted something, but you did not get it for one reason or another.
2. Feel the anger grabbing you somewhere, often in your jaw or shoulders. Where is anger focused?
3. Connect to the depth of the anger that you felt.
4. What are the sensations, where are they, and what do they want to do? Example: *My shoulders are tight and want to punch. My jaw is tight, and I want to bite or scream.*
5. As you stay with the sensations, you may want to move your shoulders or jaw.
6. As you stay with the anger, you may find that there is hurt or fear under the anger.
7. Watch the changes in physicality as you shift from anger to hurt or fear. What hurt you? What are you afraid of?
8. Go back and forth between the sensations of anger and the sensations of hurt/fear and see where you land.

IV – ANXIETY

Often, anxieties are due to some kind of separation… from self, other, the natural world, or the divine. When you are separated from yourself, you are missing your valuable essence, and thus are limited. You do not have a full deck, so to speak, so of course you are anxious.

You may feel other forms of anxiety and not know cognitively why. Anxiety could be about something in the environment that your system picks up. You may not perceive the threat. But your system is telling you about it. *Neuroception,* the term coined by Stephen Porges, PhD, refers to how our neural circuits distinguish whether stimuli are safe or dangerous. It occurs in the brain's primitive regions without conscious awareness.[3]

One client was very anxious and settled herself by smoking cigarettes. During a session, I had her move in different ways and change her breathing pattern. She reported that after the session: "When I am organized like this, I don't need to feel anxious. Thus, I don't need to smoke." She had no desire for a cigarette. When physicality is stable and supported, often, one does not need to feel anxious or to act out behaviors to calm those feelings. This can also go the other way: when some people feel settled, they may become more anxious. This can be the case when/if trauma happened during sleep or a restful state.

EX – Purpose of Habits

1. We want to keep in mind (and body) that every behavior, emotion, and habit served a purpose at some time. Otherwise, you wouldn't do it.
2. What does smoking cigarettes or your habit do for you now, or how does it make you feel? What is good about it? How does it serve you?
3. Be honest with yourself as you explore this question.
4. As you get to the root of the question, be compassionate with yourself, as you wonder if the habit is still serving you.

EX – Direction of Anxiety

1. When you begin to feel anxiety, there is often this rising up of some energy or particles inside. When someone is anxious, you see the quivering upward.
2. In contrast, the salubrious energy from the ground that goes up for deep support is going down. The overall physicality is collapsed.
3. The directions are all backward. Shift the energy and reverse the directions.
4. Let the ground support come up, and let the quiver settle down.
5. Performance anxiety is discussed in Chapter 11.

EX – Anxiety in Action

1. When I feel anxiety, I feel the little bubbles all over the front of my body.
2. I ask, *What am I anxious about?* (Not saying something clever)
3. In the past did you blurt out clever observations? (For the most part I did or do…)
4. So why are you anxious now?
5. The bubbles are a little less.
6. I watch the bubbles.
7. How would they like to move?
8. They would like to find a calming rhythm. Anxiety is a frantic, buzzing rhythm.
9. Does any image come up? (Riding on a boat in calm waters)
10. Bubbles settle a bit more.
11. I see myself knocked off center, losing footing, a very old memory. When the body is going to fall, you feel anxious.
12. Are you going to fall now? (No)
13. My system settles. The bubbles are fewer.

EX – Electric Current of Calm

People with anxiety or other fear-based conditions typically will breathe rapidly, often using the scalene muscles on the sides of the neck. This engages the sympathetic branch of the nervous system, encouraging the production of adrenaline. You can calm the nervous system with a longer *Humm* exhale that stimulates a parasympathetic response. The parasympathetic part of the nervous system facilitates

IV – ANXIETY

rest and relaxation, whereas the sympathetic part arouses fight-or-flight responses.

1. Place your hands on your kidneys in back. Your adrenal glands, on top of your kidneys, secrete adrenaline and cortisol.
2. Feel the contact, warmth, or holding—the nervous system markers for release or reset.
3. Rest your hands.
4. Make a humming sound. Any pitch. This releases nitric oxide, which provides a defense against invaders, kills viruses. Therapist and author Gabor Maté says, as a metaphor, that trauma is like a virus, a perpetrator, invading you. Trauma is the result of what happened. It lives inside and spreads.[4]
5. Now combine the two practices: hands on kidney/adrenal area and humming. An electric current of calm is possible, as your whole body buzzes.

V – FEAR

Fear is a huge emotion for many people. It so often stops wonderful ideas from coming to life—there is a fear that others will laugh, or not like or not support it. The fear cripples progress with strong physical and emotional messages. The fear circuitry in the brain includes the periaqueductal gray, which is the threat and pain detector. It is deep inside the brain above the brainstem. It activates the amygdala in the midbrain, to signal danger. People with dissociative disorders show hyperconnectivity between the periaqueductal gray and amygdala.

EX – Your Own Fear: Three Steps to Change

Fear has:

1. A body sensation (gut twist).
2. A thought process (worry).
3. A memory or imagining of something that happened in the past or may happen in the future (an accident).

V – FEAR

All three steps are included in any version of fear. All three steps must be tended to.

1. For the gut twist, bring your attention to your gut. Define the twist. What direction? What is twisting? Is there any space? Any breath? Vibrate your belly with a low-pitched sound.
2. For the worry, begin to look at the thoughts. Are they familiar? Are they really true? Are they even yours?
3. For the accident, remember that it is over, and that you survived. Because it happened once, does that mean it will happen again? Remember the idea—*That was then; this is now.*

VI – LOVE

We are told: Love is not a thought or a feeling, but the essence of who we are. We don't find love, but we can be love. Love is our life force. How easy is this to believe and embody? Why do we fear to love?

EX – Perspectives on Love

Read these well-phrased quotes and see how they touch you.

> "Love is simply the name for the desire and pursuit of the whole. Love is born into every human being; it calls back the halves of our original nature together; it tries to make one out of two and heal the wound of human nature."
>
> —*Plato*

VI – LOVE

"And still after all this time the sun never says to Earth,
you owe me. Look what happens with a love like that;
it lights the whole sky."

—*Hafiz*

"...we must begin to love in order not to fall ill."

—*Sigmund Freud*

"Love is the great force in the universe.
Heartbeat of the moral cosmos."

—*Martin Luthur King, Jr*

"The greatest act of love is to be present to somebody."

—*Thich Nhat Hanh*

EX – Chemicals of Love

1. Dopamine, the reward and motivational chemical, gets released when you feel thankful, complete something, listen to music. And, of course, when you tap your smartphone.
2. Serotonin, a mood stabilizer, gets released when you do deeper breathing, run, or swim vigorously, and, for some people, meditate.

3. Endorphins, which remove pain and make you feel positive, are released when you dance, exercise, meditate, laugh, or sometimes when you get injured (to not feel the pain).
4. Oxytocin, the love hormone, gets released when you hug, hold hands, have healthy relationships, or when a baby is with a loving mother or caregiver. Sue Carter, PhD, Distinguished University Research Scientist at the Kinsey Institute, describes oxytocin as the biological core of what it means to be human. Her research led to the discovery of the relationship between social behavior and oxytocin, and she examined mechanisms through which oxytocin pathways help to explain both positive social experiences and physical wellness.[5] And the research by Donnalea Goelz, PhD, has shown that 90 minutes of somatic interventions (exercises that include body and mind), done once a week for three weeks, can elevate oxytocin levels.[6]

EX – Love Each Other?

As you read this next EX, what thoughts, feelings, or sensations come up for you?

>What makes a good American
>What do you have to be
>Am I a good American
>Let's take a look and see
>I like democracy
>I am for equality
>I stand up for my rights
>But do I stand up for yours?

VI – LOVE

We learned this song in the second grade (seven years old). It is called the brotherhood song. I loved it. I felt moved by it. I felt proud to sing it. I stood up tall and proud to be an American and to care about others. I thought it was a great song. My heart lifted and expanded to include myself and those around me.

Later that day in the schoolyard, my friends and I were talking about the songs we were singing. I remember saying how I loved the brotherhood song and thought it was so wonderful.

My friends laughed and made fun of me. They totally disagreed with me. When my friends said the song was stupid and meaningless, I was shattered, collapsed—a bubble burst. I didn't understand why they didn't see how wonderful this song was and how important the question…I stand up for my rights, but do I stand up for yours? I mean, really stand up, like fight and defend, if necessary. That question continues to live with me. How much do I stand up for yours? From second grade.[7]

CHAPTER 9

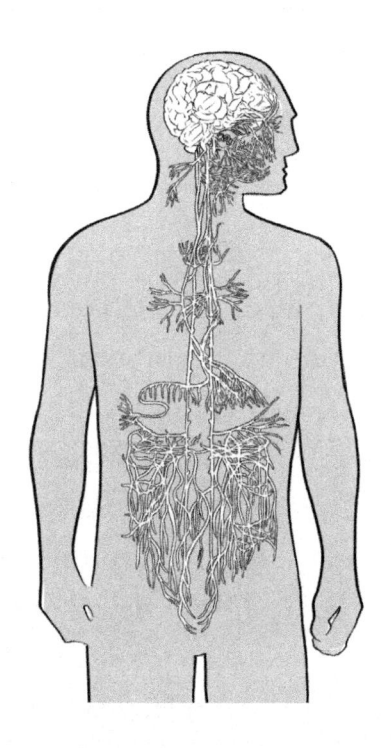

THE VAGUS NERVE AND THE POLYVAGAL THEORY

I – INTRODUCTION TO THE VAGUS NERVE

The vagus nerve, cranial nerve X or 10—the longest nerve in the body—has more than one main branch. Originally called "the wanderer," it was until recently considered to be one rambling nerve extending from the head (cranium) to the abdomen. Dr. Stephen Porges introduced the term "polyvagal" because there are in fact two definable and recognizable branches (ventral and dorsal) of this key nerve. The Polyvagal Theory (PVT) developed by Porges helps us understand the functional and adaptive nature of the vagus nerve in response to the environment, and particularly to danger.[1]

The vagus nerve is literally the captain of the parasympathetic nervous system, overseeing a vast range of crucial functions, communicating nerve impulses to every organ in your body. When you have a strong emotion or see something awful (trigger warning) like a car accident, the belly tightens. The vagus nerve has 80 percent of its nerve fibers going from belly to brain. And only 20 percent from brain to belly. That tells us that the system really wants to know what is happening in your body. The PVT traces the evolutionary relationship

I – INTRODUCTION TO THE VAGUS NERVE

of the autonomic nervous system with instinctual and social behavior. The responses to the environment range from determining that it's safe to dangerous to life-threatening. Or put more simply: okay, not okay, really not okay. Where is your breaking point? When are you not okay? When does your nervous system jump into high gear? Everybody goes at some point.

EX – Vagus Nerve Functions

- Reduces inflammation.
- Initiates regulation.
- Helps make memories.
- Controls your heart rate.
- Tells your brain how you are feeling.

We can see these functions in action in the following EXploracises.

EXPLORACISES

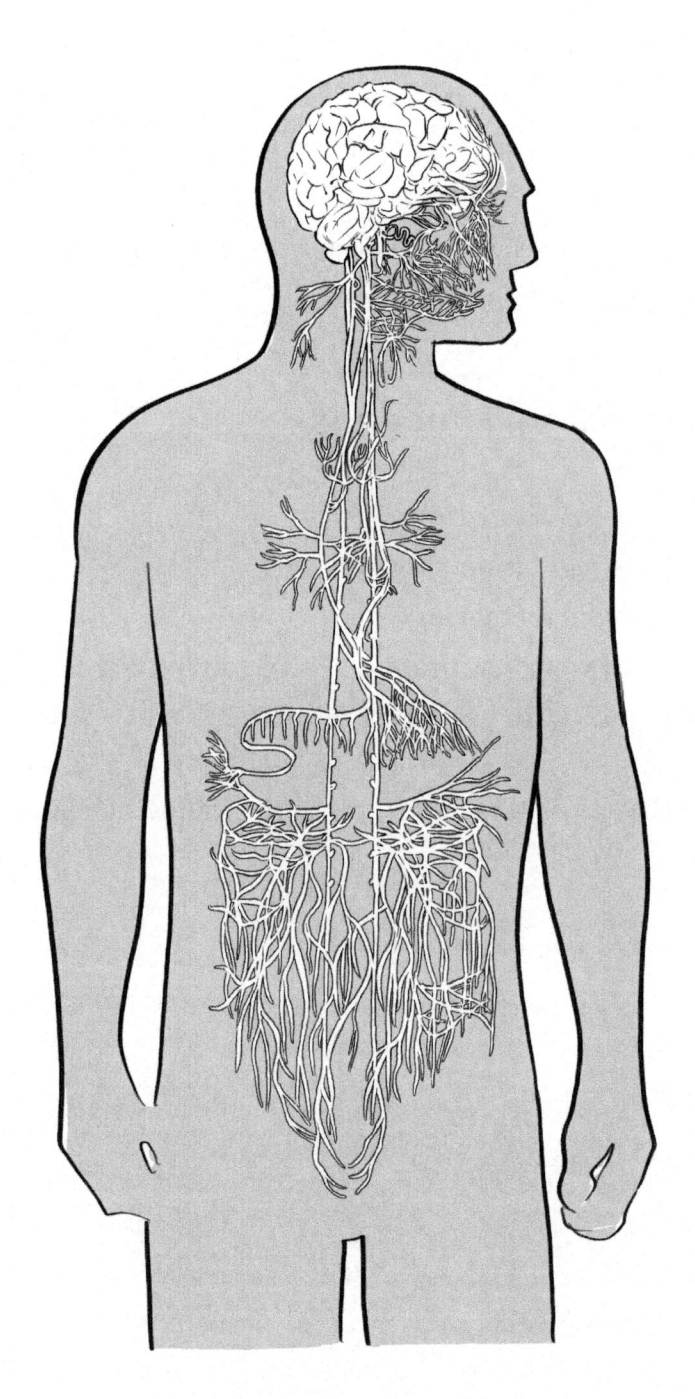

Vagus Nerve

II – POLYVAGAL EXPLORACISES

The PVT reframes the interpretation of overwhelm from *we have a permanent condition of something* to *we are responding to our environment, real or perceived.* Overwhelm is a state-related phenomenon. If we perceive the environment as dangerous, then we respond with fear and a sympathetic state. Instead of calling it stress, you realize that you perceive danger, and your nervous system is responding accordingly.

The PVT recognizes the connection between social behavior and the autonomic nervous system. It links sociality to homeostatic function. One example of this is a study that was done with Ed Tronick's still-face experiment, which goes as follows: A caregiver enjoys an interaction with a baby, then the caregiver looks away, the baby gets upset, and then the caregiver comes back in contact. The PVT team explored the tone of voice that the caregiver came back with. They found that when the caregiver used a prosodic, melodic voice, the baby became much calmer, and the baby's heart rate dropped by 10 beats per minute. This shows that a ventral vagal social engagement expression can signal safety and help calm the autonomic nervous system. The system co-regulates to feel safe enough to be with another.[2]

EX – Physiology of Polyvagal

1. Ventral vagal: When you feel safe, notice what happens in your body. Perhaps there is more homeostasis with a settling breath, ease in the muscular system, and an ability to expand to connection and ask for help if you need it. You can feel safe with gentle, attuned touch, or when you are balanced over your feet so you don't fall, or by recognizing that the space around you is not threatening. Who are you when you feel safe enough and trust that it is safe enough to be who you are? We need to belong to survive.
2. Sympathetic: Notice what happens when you sense danger. There is an immediate alertness or hyper-alertness, or muscular tightening, as your body wonders and seeks where the danger is. Breathing is faster, and blood flows to the muscles and away from internal organs, creating "butterflies." This prepares you to protect yourself from the danger.
3. Dorsal vagal: If the danger continues and escalates, the situation may be life-threatening. You may feel helpless. Your systems shut down, you are frozen with fear, and the body is numb. This can show as rigidity or flaccidity, as both are numbed states.

Recognize that these three states can shift from one to another quite quickly. All systems have gradations and degrees of intensity. For example, a functional freeze will allow certain organs, often the heart, to have no feeling while the rest of you moves through life.[3] Or your sympathetic system will emerge when there is danger, but it will also get you to the gym.

EX – Polyvagal Muscular Pulls to Explore

1. Ventral vagal is the following: Ease in facial muscles, softer eye gaze, slight smile, head is freely balancing.
2. Sympathetic is the following: Muscles firm up and are ready for action in arms and legs, direct eye gaze, with narrow focus to find the danger.
3. Dorsal vagal is the following: Muscles are either stiff and rigid or flaccid and collapsed, eyes often staring with a faraway gaze to nowhere.

EX – Speed of Polyvagal States When Walking

1. Ventral vagal: Movement is appropriate for the moment, and generally slow and purposeful. Feet in contact with the ground.
2. Sympathetic: Moves like electricity or a fire burning kiln-dried wood. It ignites fast, travels fast, and is hard to stop. Feet pulled up off the ground.
3. Dorsal vagal: Moves slowly or not at all. Like with green wood, it is hard to get a fire going. Feet heavy into the ground.

EX – Bones in Response to Danger

New research suggests that bones are involved in a fight-or-flight response. The research revealed that the skeleton releases osteocalcin, which travels through the bloodstream to affect the biological functions of the pancreas, brain, muscles, and other organs. The researchers found in mice (when threatened) and humans (for public speaking) that almost immediately after the brain recognizes danger, it instructs the skeleton to flood the bloodstream with the bone-derived hormone osteocalcin, which is needed to turn on the fight-or-flight response. According to the study's senior investigator, "In bony vertebrates, the acute stress response is not possible without osteocalcin."[4] This is interesting when we remember our biotensegrity model. There is constant interaction between the bones and soft tissue. Responses to danger would not be muscular or hormonal only, but would include the structural aspects also. Bones are living tissue, not just solid blocks.

Next time you experience any type of overwhelm or danger, remember that your bones are part of the process, not just adrenaline and cortisol.

III – HUMANUAL POLYVAGAL SMILE

1. *Start with a small smile:*
   Feel the corners of your mouth extend to your outer ears. Like a band across your lower face.
2. *Smile again:*
   Take that energetic band inward toward the interior of your head, so that from the back of your throat you feel a slight opening to your middle ears in the interior of your head. It is a stretch from middle ear to middle ear.
3. *You smile again:*
   This time allow the smile to resonate up to your eyes. Often a slight opening can happen—a moment of excitement, a feeling of something elevated. The circular muscles around your eyes expand a bit.
   With that there is often a breath. Stay with that for a moment or two.

4. *Then again – Slight smile:*
   This time drop your awareness down to your neck and notice how the smile feels in your throat, your voice, your larynx.
5. *Another smile:*
   Bring your attention to your breath, lungs, and heart.
   Spread out through your chest to your arms to your fingertips, as you raise your arms up and out to the side.
6. *And one more – slight smile:*
   This time drop your attention down to see how the smile affects your belly. Then travel down mentally and energetically through your legs to the ground.
7. With practice, you can do all the steps quickly in succession, almost all at once, allowing yourself to experience the HUMANUAL Polyvagal Smile—a full self/body event. Relish any and all small adjustments and discoveries each time you do it.[5]

III – HUMANUAL POLYVAGAL SMILE

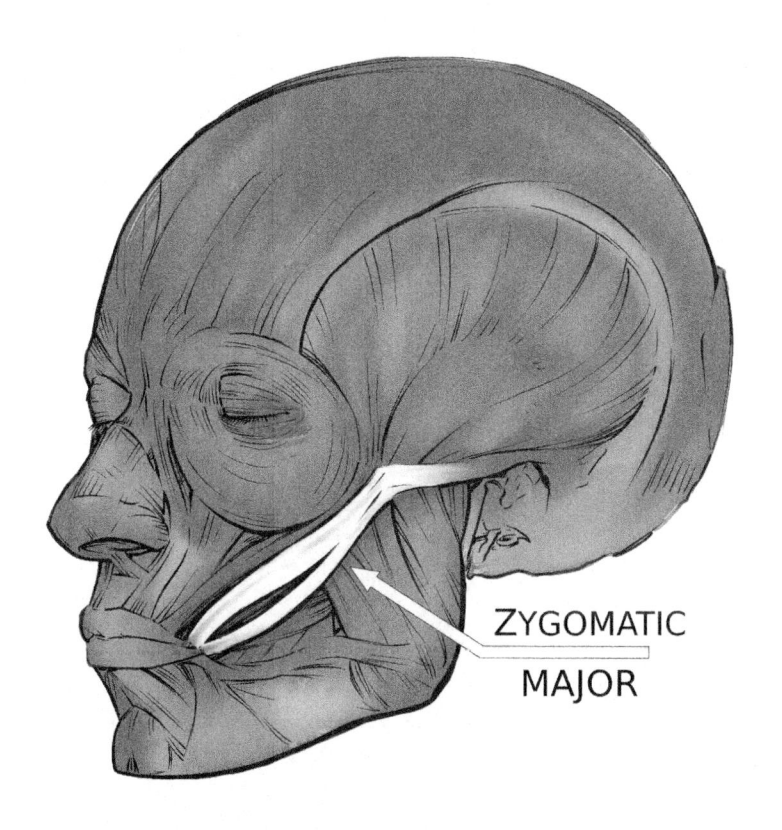

Zygomatic Muscle

CHAPTER 10

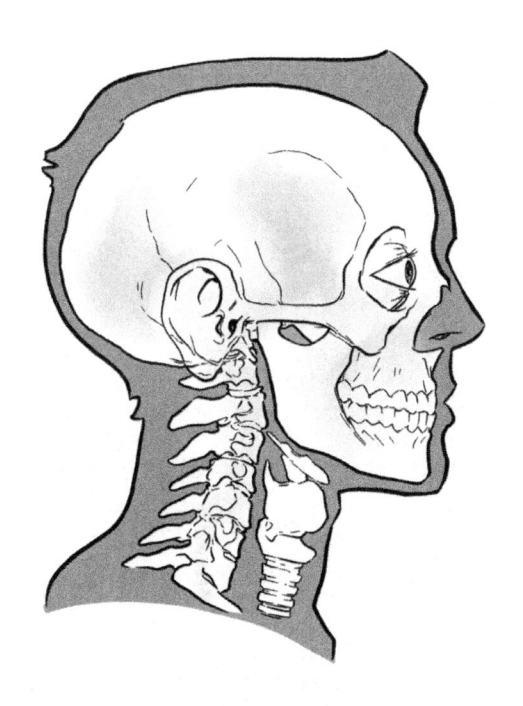

TRAUMA

I – INTRODUCTION TO TRAUMA

EX – Considering Trauma

Trauma is a popular word these days. It is overused in both directions:

1. Some people think they have trauma but don't. *Oh, I saw a movie last night, and it traumatized me.* No, it upset you.
2. Some people say all is well. *No trauma here. Nothing ever happened to me.* But then if someone cuts in front of them while driving, they go into a rage. Clearly, something other than the driver is causing the rage.
3. Those who think they have trauma may not, and those who don't think they have trauma might warrant a closer look. We all fall both ways sometimes. Which category do you fall into most often?

I – INTRODUCTION TO TRAUMA

EX – Trauma Definitions

See if any of these descriptions of trauma apply to you.

- Simply put: Something bad happened, and no one was there to help, and you were left with some unpleasant reminders such as pathways embedded in your nervous system or patterns in your body. That can happen slowly, developmentally, as you are growing, or it can be one big, difficult, shocking event at any time of life that dysregulates your nervous system.
- Sometimes the environment as you were growing up was not supportive or did not give you what you needed. There was misattunement between you and your caregiver, so you had to create behaviors that sort of gave you what you needed, as a substitute. This allowed you to survive. If the early environment did not support your worthiness, you will constantly try to prove that you are worthy, even as an adult.
- If one parent was depressed, a child might always be smiling and trying to cheer the parent up. That smile becomes an adaptive pattern. It hides the emotional trauma. Sometimes we had to shut off what was most real and alive to us and create unconscious adaptive patterns. Now, most of us do not need these survival patterns anymore. They are not serving us.
- We all have many of these patterns that we do not recognize. They are lingering effects of trauma. We create adaptations to "hide" the trauma. Remember that every dysfunctional behavior or what we now call a problem once served a purpose for our survival.

EX – Trauma Is a Wound—Often a Wound You Cannot See

Nobody gets through life without a few bumps. Some bumps are worse than others. Remember a time when:

1. You have a small bump or accident, and you brush it off. No big deal.
2. Other times you bump into something, and it hurts. You are wounded.
3. Later, the event may be over, but the black-and-blue mark is still there, or the broken bone that you can see and must patiently support to heal.
4. Some wounds you cannot see. They get imprinted in the nervous system as a lack of regulation. You see or feel the symptoms or results of the dysregulation, but you don't see the dysregulation itself.
5. Perhaps this is what makes some trauma so elusive. You cannot see it, nor can others see it just by looking. They need to ask you questions. But you know something is off or wrong. So, you also need to ask yourself questions.

II – TRAUMA EXPLORACISES

My early years as a dance and movement teacher were devoted to discovering how the body moves most efficiently, how to not get injured, and how to recover if you did get injured. I looked for an ideal formula that allowed freedom of motion and breath. As I learned how the physical body best functions, I was able to help others find their way back to our innate internal organization of wellbeing with synchronized embodiment. A kind of primordial unity of structure. The knee bends one way and not the other.

The structure or "design" itself works, but not everybody is able to make use of it. What is in the way? What makes a person choose their ingrained pattern over the ancient, innate, integrative pattern I show them? That is how I discovered trauma. Certain emotional and adaptive patterns pull people away from the internal organization of health and wellbeing. It may look like part of yourself is missing.

My task has always been to be aware of the potential of everybody, that resides deep inside under the traumatic patterns. I do not focus on "getting rid of the trauma." I help you connect to your underlying somatic blueprint, the internal organization, that balances life energy and resolves symptoms that are imprinted patterns from your history. You don't want to erase trauma or relive it, but you want to connect to yourself through the network of the traumatic manifestations. That is done with self-compassion and wisdom. If you have an extensive trauma history, or if many overwhelming emotions come up for you, you may want to do some of the EXs in the company of a therapist.

EX – Physical Manifestations of Trauma

All trauma affects your head (thinking, constant judging thoughts), heart (emotions, pain of relationship), and/or belly (gut feeling). Let's start with that.

1. Touch the top of your head with both hands. What do you notice, if anything? Maybe one side has more energy or activity than the other.
2. Put both hands on the chest area on top of your heart. What do you notice, if anything? Maybe depression in or pushing out?
3. Touch the top of your belly with both hands. What do you notice, if anything? Maybe over- or under-activity?
4. Notice any change at all in your cognitive, emotional, or physical body.

11 – TRAUMA EXPLORACISES

EX – Overwhelm Can Happen Two Ways

1. By your emotional overload, and the results of your traumatic experience.
2. Or, if you are on a healing journey, the moment the trauma shifts can be overwhelming. The system is not used to that kind of energy.
3. Overwhelm can come from either. Be gentle with yourself. Detect slight overwhelm, and stay with that. Remain at the edge. Tracking skills are important here. (See Chapter 3.)

EX – Numb

Parts of us go numb because we are not able to feel what is there. We either don't want to or can't—possibly from pain, or loss of function. We get body amnesia.

1. If you feel numb in one place, see what surrounds it. Where is numb? Where is feeling?
2. Where do they meet? What happens there? Come to your own edge of where they meet. Describe it.
3. There is no such thing as not feeling anything, unless you are unconscious or dead. Your belly has feeling. Your chest and throat have feeling. The bottoms of your feet have feeling. Don't make it into what it "should" feel like. What is there? Work with what is there, for new somatic mobilization.

EX – Trauma and Healing

It's not about healing the body. It's about discovering the need for the symptoms in all realms: emotional, physical, and spiritual.

1. What happened to you, so that you need these symptoms? How did you feel?
2. When you no longer need the symptoms, healing and wholeness are evident. What would that be like?
3. Trauma often does not come back as a memory but as a behavior or reaction to present circumstances. Can you name some behaviors and reactions of yours?
4. When you understand clearly what has happened, and what you are doing, you can have a clue as to how you might proceed for healing.
5. How would you like to move forward, following what matters to you?

EX – Trauma and Symptoms

Trauma is not the event itself, but the response to life that is left. Unprocessed, overwhelming events that were not completed or metabolized create symptoms in the present time. If you had an experience of overwhelm or trauma that is stuck in a somatic pattern, you will need to offer conditions for change. Imprints do not recognize how much time has passed since the event. It doesn't matter how old you were when it happened. They feel like very present and valid parts of yourself that are still believing that those scenarios are real. The undigested movement and behaviors show up now as symptoms.

II – TRAUMA EXPLORACISES

As you metabolize and digest, you get your life energy and essence back, and the energy of the symptoms gets repurposed to work for you and not against you. Life can then move forward. You do not want to relive, express, erase, punch pillows, or deny trauma, but instead use the physicality to connect to the self through the network of trauma:

1. See, feel, and sense what the trauma is doing, saying, and believing, right now in this present moment—the moment you choose to belong to, and recognize and take for reality.
2. Essential bodily functions such as skin temperature, digestion, blood pressure, heart rate, and immune physiology related to daily life get set aside or stressed when stress physiology takes over. The digestive system is often the first place to dysregulate when trauma happens. Are you noticing any symptoms in these areas?
3. What are you actually doing? Being angry, saying thank-you, proving you're right, judging, or enjoying life?
4. Does what you are doing match what you are intending to do?
5. Can you learn to be present to powerful energy? Or is one of your symptoms a kind of weakness?
6. Do you want more options in life?
7. Some people have symptoms and do not know why. One possibility that might apply: Versed is a drug used as an anesthetic for surgery. It does not allow a memory to be created in the mind. When the body has a memory and the mind doesn't, it confuses the system and can interfere with healing. The body remembers the pain, and the mind does not. This creates confusion.

EX – Objectifying the Body

1. Do you tend to objectify your body?
2. Do you say "it" is hurting instead of "my shoulder" is hurting?
3. Or, even more distant, do you say "the" shoulder is hurting?
4. The lack of a compassionate and nurturing self—a self that instead objectifies the body—can make the trauma response less available for processing.

EX – Hardwired to Heal

The lingering effects of trauma can be transmuted. Food waste transforms into compost, into life-giving soil. Survival impulses can support the human composting, developing black-gold soil. What happened is over. Many somatic therapeutic processes can lead you to this healing transformation.

1. Remember, we will get through this. We will get through this story, even though feelings get triggered.
2. It will take as long as it takes to evaporate. It has a finite shelf life. It won't bother you forever, in the same way. It can move to the back burner.
3. You have what it takes to heal. You are hardwired to get through this. You have fortitude to endure. You know how to do this.
4. We are geared for wellbeing, but the deeper, longtime breaches often will not change without some attention and awareness, and the help of another. Most traumas happened in relationship, and need to be healed in relationship.

III – ANATOMICAL FACTS RELATED TO TRAUMATIC RESPONSES

Trauma responses change the innate pattern of how the body functions. In this section you will learn more or review your existing knowledge about how bones, fascia, and muscles are put together and how they move most efficiently. When there is some kind of physical pain, simply put, it is from 1) disease, 2) injury (physical or emotional), or 3) misuse. Most are familiar with 1 and 2, but very few talk about 3, as it is not taught in school or anywhere else (explained in Chapter 1).

Main categories of trauma responses:

- A thwarted fight response often shows up in arms. The person wanted to fight with their arms, but for one reason or another, they were not able to complete the urge to hit, punch, protect, or push.
- A thwarted flight response often shows up in legs. The person wanted to flee with their legs, but for one reason or another, they were not able to complete the urge to run, move away, or escape.

- A freeze response is a combination of fight and flight. The person was not able to fight or flee, and maybe had to freeze; either way, they are stuck, often with limited movement.
- A collapse response is often manifest in the central torso. It is similar to the freeze but has a droopy, helpless quality, without stiffness.
- A thwarted emotional response often shows up as a collapsed chest or heart.
- A thwarted fawning or people-pleasing response often shows up as leaning forward and trying to connect.

Starting at the top:

EX – Head

1. Find the top of your spine:
   It is halfway to the center of your head from each ear.
   It is halfway to the center of your head from the front and back. The top of your spine meets the cranial base.
   When there has been trauma, often, the head is not balanced on top of the spine. This may be from some kind of impact, looking for something, away from something, or a fear, startle, or shame response. The classic startle pattern has the head dropped back and down and pulled in, as the shoulders come up. The classic shame response is the head dropped forward and gaze averted.
2. Bring attention to the top of your spine:
   This is somatic head balancing. The concept of "somatic" includes mind and the constantly adjusting living body.

III – ANATOMICAL FACTS RELATED TO TRAUMATIC RESPONSES

Balancing is finding or allowing the place of least resistance. When the body is balanced, it is not held, stiffened, or rigid; it is constantly adjusting to the thoughts, emotions, and environment. Your head certainly wants to do this.

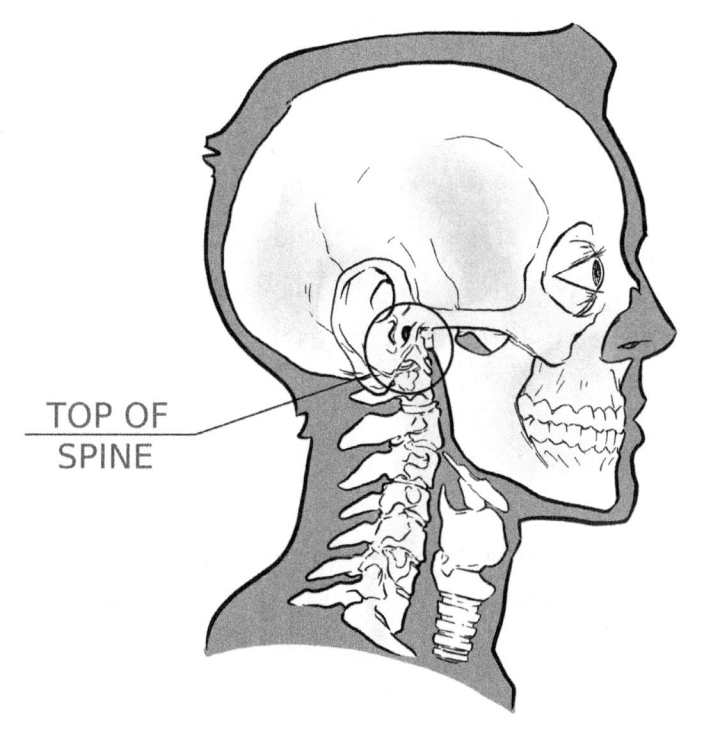

Top of the spine

3. The weight of your head:
   Holding your head back and down puts weight on the nerve channel in your spine. The vertebrae have a bony mass and a cushion disk, and a channel for nerves. You want to put weight on the bony mass, not the nerve channel behind it. When your head is dropped down on your spine, your spine compresses, and the muscles on both sides constrict and restrict the movement of the spine. The internal organs are then

compromised, creating further dis-harmony or dis-ease. In order to restore ease in the torso, the head must find freedom at the top of the spine.

Your head dropped back with constriction is a sympathetic response—the system is activated and ready for defense. Your head balanced on top of your spine is ventral vagal, ready for social engagement. Your head dropped or collapsed forward or backward is often a shutdown. When the head is not dropped on the spine in any way, shape, or form, the spine can pulse itself to lengthen, and the vertebrae and ribs expand in all directions (360 degrees). We then feel the life force and pulse of living, and that has the potential to carry us into forward motion.

EX – Arm Movement

Your arms have four major joints, not three, as most people think, counting the wrist, elbow, and shoulder joint. But in truth, you must include as the fourth joint the place where the collarbone meets the sternum: the sternoclavicular joint (SC). If you move or rotate your collarbone, you will see that your arm moves, showing us that this is functionally a major arm joint. I once worked with a female trombone player, and she was not able to get the full range of slide length for sound. After I taught her where her arm began, she was able to extend her instrument to its full slide potential.

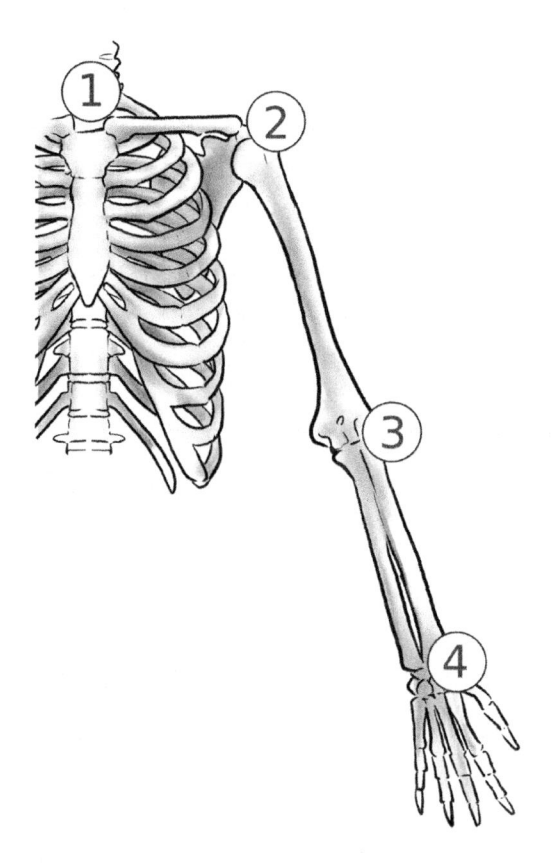

III – ANATOMICAL FACTS RELATED TO TRAUMATIC RESPONSES

Sternoclavicular Joint at 1

Feel the difference.

1. Move your arm from your shoulder joint.
2. Explore moving your arm from the sternoclavicular joint, by putting your hand on your collarbone, and finding the movement that is available to you.
3. Feel the difference between the two.

Notice how step 2 is tied to your mouth, neck, voice, and breathing. If your trauma involved not being able to speak, which causes a tight throat, this practice can begin to help you find the words that got buried or lost in the moment or moments of overwhelm. Also, moving from the SC joint has the potential to dismantle some of the holding of the shame posture; the tendency for having your head dropped down and gaze turned away can rebalance. Finding movement at some of these less-used joints can break up general bracing patterns. As the changes occur, one can digest each small change and the emotions, sensations, and feelings associated with that position.

EX – Shoulder Blades

Shoulder blades are mobile. They are not attached to the spine or ribs. They glide on your back. They are movable, and they are available to help you push something away, or to embrace something.

1. Stand near a wall. Push through your arm against the wall, one then the other arm.
2. Feel the movability of your shoulder blade. Can you enjoy the feeling of the push?
3. Think of a time you wanted to push but were not able to. When you push, does it feel good? Or scary (like something bad will happen)?
4. Stay with that and see what comes up.
5. The free movement of your shoulder blades is strongly tied to the ease and efficiency of your breath. Does a tight shoulder inhibit breath or does held breath cause a tight shoulder? Both are possible. Changing your use can invite a change in the emotion held in the joint of your upper arm and shoulder blade. You don't want your shoulder blades sitting heavy on your ribs.
6. Move your shoulders forward and back, one at a time.
7. Move one forward and one back at the same time.

III – ANATOMICAL FACTS RELATED TO TRAUMATIC RESPONSES

8. Do small rotations or circles while one is forward and the other is back.
   Reverse direction.
9. Any change or freedom in your jaw? Many odd mouth habits or pulls involve the shoulders, because the top shoulder muscles go up the neck to the lower jaw.
10. In the wake of a traumatic event, the whole shoulder girdle (scapula and collarbone) can end up drooped far forward or pulled back military-style (the old pull-your-shoulders-back idiom). Neither of these fits our anatomical structure. Picture your shoulder girdle like a yoke that is sitting evenly balanced over your spine. Try moving it far forward, then far back, then find the middle, which will include a widening across your shoulders, and probably a breath.

EX – Elbow Joint

The elbow bends and rotates the lower arm. A bent elbow that is pulled in is often done to protect, when being more aggressive was not possible.

1. Lift arms over your head.
2. Bring your elbows down fast, as you bend your knees and breathe out.
3. Repeat, this time coming down strong and saying HA!
4. This helps release pent-up anger and frustration you were unable to previously express.

EXPLORACISES

EX – Spine

1. Lie down on your back, knees bent and feet flat, with a small folded towel under your head, so your head is not compressed into your spine.
2. Become aware of any pressure or tensing in your spine, from the pelvic floor to the top of your spine.
   The dilemma: The spine wants to be elongated, but our emotional life needs to respond with a contraction or pulling in to hide or protect, so the structure is compromised. When you are crunched down or collapsed, see how you breathe or see how easy or difficult it is to move.
3. See if you can allow more length in your spine, thus releasing the pressure and allowing more space in your internal organs, including allowing fuller breath.
4. Repeat the release of pressure and see if there are any words that want to be said:
   "See me." "I want to expand." Any movement that goes along with the words?
   A musician hears music in their head to get ready to play, and the body must make movements to play this music. It is the same for all of us. Our thoughts and words have a body expression. My spine moves differently when I say "I love you" than when I say "I hate you." The body movement is the mind's thoughts. They are one and the same. Put this together for yourself. Become aware of the movement of your spine.

III – ANATOMICAL FACTS RELATED TO TRAUMATIC RESPONSES

5. Undulate your spine as you lie on the floor. Drop into collapse and then lengthen up. Move like a jellyfish in your spine. Try it with your hand first—expand, and then dome your palm up as you contract and bring your fingers together. Find a rhythm. Then add your spine.

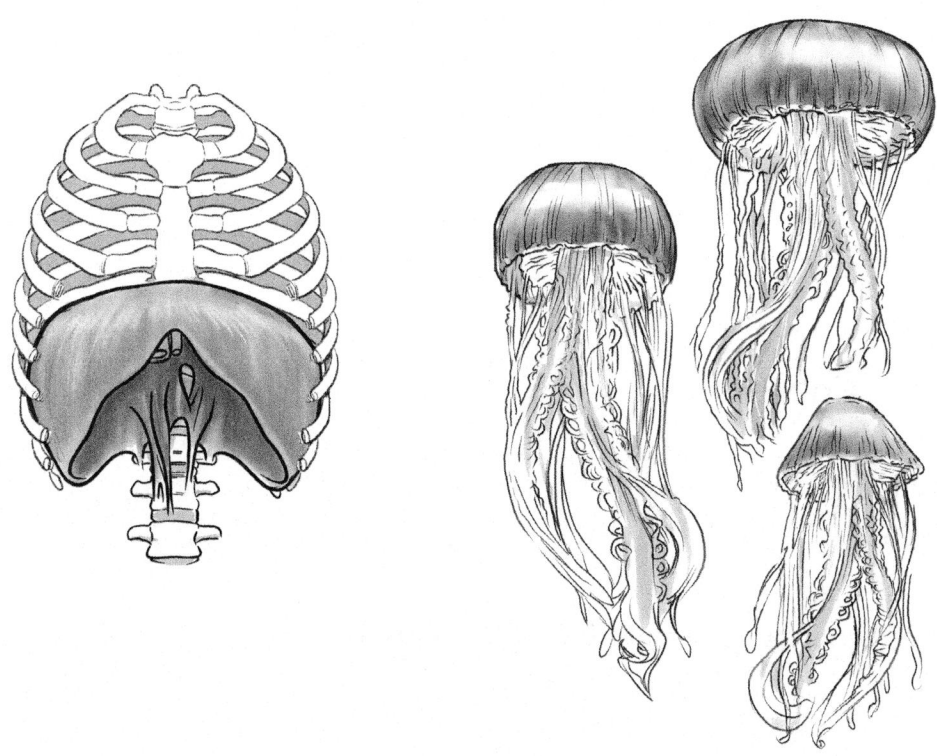

Diaphragm and Jellyfish

EX – Pelvis

1. With any kind of sexual abuse or trauma, there will most likely be holding in the genital, pelvic, and buttock area. If you are in a safe place or with a trusted person, you can explore tending to some of the pelvic holdings.
2. Move your pelvis in figure 8s. Both directions. If the pulls are uneven, gently explore and coax the place where there is less movement.
3. Gently rock your pelvis slightly forward and back, about a quarter inch. Notice the different pulls on both sides and/or restrictions.
4. Many inner pelvic floor muscles will need to adjust as the pelvis rebalances itself.

EX – Knees

Your knee only bends forward for movement. When you hyperextend or lock your knees back, you are trying to bend them backward. It will not work and might cause pain. Children often lock their knees when they are anxious or not liking what is going on, a kind of "NO."

1. As you stand, feel how much pressure is at the back of your knees.
2. Slowly let the pressure release.
3. Allow your heels to drop into the ground to help this.
4. Do not just immediately bend your knees to change the locked position.

III – ANATOMICAL FACTS RELATED TO TRAUMATIC RESPONSES

EX – Rest, Even for a Second

1. Notice that with an overwhelming event, or even after deep work, thoughts and emotions can be all over the place. For some, their nervous system is firing fast, bouncing off the walls like the silver balls in a pinball machine.
2. *Whoa,* stop.
3. Offer each pinball a place to rest. One by one, give them an invitation and an opportunity to rest. Ask: Are you tired? Would you like to rest?
4. Then picture a cushion or soft bed, and imagine that you curl up and rest your whole self.
5. Rest for a moment, and make it conscious for at least a second. The body, mind, and spirit can rest and be supported.
6. Recognize that movement and rest are the way of the universe. If you don't rest, it will come to you. You will be forced to rest.
7. Rest not just outer body movement but inner thoughts and emotions, even for a second.

Yes, it can be hard to rest. How can we really rest when there is culturally induced prejudice, racial trauma, and mass killing that is very real? The idea is absolutely ridiculous that only certain races or people deserve comfortable lives. And even more ridiculous to witness some striving to become trillionaires, while so many are starving. Those of us who have enough must take extra care to not fall into the well-worn paradigms of superiority.

The main race is the human race. We are all winners. Please, no more forcing Indigenous people to give up their innate, native wisdom. No more racially profiling dark-skinned people. No more persecution because of religious beliefs. No more killing just because you can. The patterns are deeply sown. Ancestral trauma is real. Our patterns get passed down in many forms, and they can affect us in ways we don't even notice.

In addition to trauma, we inherit wisdom from our ancestors. Do what you can to see the human race. Many philosophers, astrologers, and prophets have said that we are moving from individual consciousness to group consciousness with the shifts in the precessional cycle of the equinoxes. Our 24,000-year precessional cycle is most likely due to the Earth's movement around a binary star, which many believe is Sirius, the brightest star in our sky. We measure this cycle by observing the shifts in the constellation rising before sunrise at the spring equinox in the northern hemisphere (the autumn equinox in the southern hemisphere). The shifts in the ages occur approximately every 2,000 years and bring changes to our cultural paradigms and ways of being. We are now moving into the Age of Aquarius associated with harmony, openness to diversity, and collaboration in community.

Many cultures have their own version of this phenomenon. Ancient Hindu legend and cosmology detailed the Yuga cycles—an ever-circling ascending culture (celebrating our humanity) and a descending culture (forgetting our highest ideals). These cycles chart the evolution of our human consciousness. We are currently at the end of a 6,000-year period of the Kali Yuga, the lowest level of consciousness in the cycle, characterized by being mired in disconnection, separation from each other and from Source. We are at the cusp of moving into a period of ascending consciousness and into greater unity consciousness. These cycles may also help explain how the ancient Egyptians, Mayans, and others had advanced cultural civilizations thousands of years ago. History is not linear, it is cyclical or spiraling.

Change is happening, slowly but surely. Many of the EXploracises can help reduce past limiting beliefs. Heaven and Earth in synchronized embodiment is meant for all. "We are all divine beings having an earthly experience." This quote is attributed to French philosopher Pierre Teilhard de Chardin in The Joy of Kindness (1993) by Robert J. Furey, but many say that Greek philosophers used the expression long ago.

Can we rest and free our body, mind, and spirit to release us from this culturally induced trauma coma and come home to our divine blessings and power? Despite our traumas and difficulty, evolution continues, exhausting and/or energizing. We are receiving waves from the galactic current and solar flares. Our world and the movement of the planets will change beyond our wildest dreams. It's not letting up. There is no turning back. No dress rehearsal. The consciousness in everything is here as part of the change—exhilarating, deeply soothing, painfully sobering, and sometimes completely joyous.

CHAPTER 11

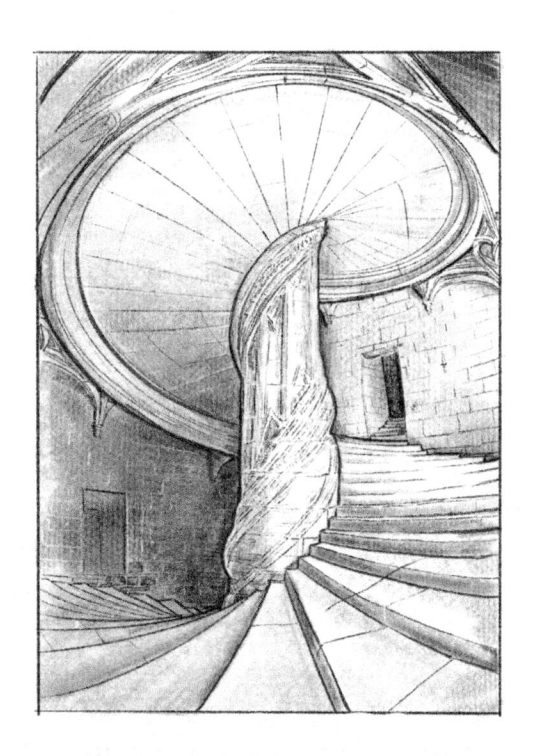

PERFORMANCE

I – INTRODUCTION TO PERFORMANCE

I had a dream a few years ago that helped me find my signature style to work with performers. The Dream:

I was in a club, and Frank Sinatra was singing. When Frank sang "My Way," he looked at me, and I felt a very deep connection to him and the song. He mentioned it was a Don Costa arrangement. Don was acutely aware of some kind of sadness or trauma in life, and he conveyed that through music in a profound way. His arrangements did that for Sinatra.

As Sinatra sang, he was able to emotionally embrace his own experiences and transport his listeners, by embodying the story as a singer, actor, and dancer. People felt he was singing to them alone and their life experiences. In my dream he was singing to me and conveying the full range of human emotion. Then, the song "My Way" was mine.

Performance includes the following: your environment; the universal forces of gravitational support; the wonders of the fascial system; and the total absorption in what you are doing. Many people

I – INTRODUCTION TO PERFORMANCE

are nervous before they go on stage because "it's me and all my anxieties," but once they're on stage, they are absorbed in what they are doing. In that place of wholeness, there is no anxiety. The performance, the preparation, the physicality of the oneness, the support from the ground, all come together as one experience.

It takes practice. Practice does not make perfect. Practice makes permanent. As a performer, when you connect to the environment through the wholeness of the physicality, environment, and emotional system, in that moment there is less difference between the performer and the audience, me and you. The heart, body, and soul are the connectors. We are moved by performances of that caliber.

The Universal oneness that I know, combined with my dream of Sinatra, allowed me to put it together: the oneness, the music, the rhythm, the depth, the emotion, the heart, the fear patterns. All in one moment, a gift—the gift that is freely given all the time, though we just don't see it. I'm here to help people see it. And I will continue to do that. Thanks, Frank.

"Don't despair. Regroup."

—*Frank Sinatra*

EX – Support, Suspension, and Breath in Performance

1. Physicality: Support from the ground. Suspension from the top of the spine. Breath is three-dimensional.
2. Speaking: Support for my voice. Suspension, in my throat. Breathing, while speaking with long exhales and fluid shape changes.
3. Thinking: Support for my thoughts. Suspended and not rigid, so they can change. Breath gives time to think.
4. Emotion: Support for my emotions. Suspension to hold them. Breath so they move through.

II – ACTING

Telling stories has been a pastime for humankind forever, as it is a connection between Heaven, humans, and Earth. Ancient cultures told stories of the gods and faraway planetary cosmology as they were acting out mystical rituals to pass on to future generations. We are all actors, and we all play roles. We all have chosen archetypes that we manifest in daily life to tell our story. We have our favorite characters that we play well and ones that we don't play well. Some play angels and some play villains. As an actor, and in life, you want to be ready for anything. So when the moment changes and something gets your attention, you can respond to the moment of transition. Acting is motion and emotion in synchronized embodiment, not a body but a person in their entirety, connected to Heaven and Earth.

EX – Actors (and we?) want to:

- Experience every word and gesture.
- Know that life can be upsetting.
- Know that life is emotional.
- Go where no one wants to go, and show others it can be done. Good actors do this.
- Listen to the other like forest animals, like your life depends on it.
- Need each other to play the game.
- Tell stories that must be told.
- Stella Adler, master acting teacher, said, "It's not in the lines you say, but in the life behind it."

EX – Styles of Acting

There are many styles of acting training. It is educational work that often has therapeutic benefits. Actors must include their whole psychophysical selves, as they need to learn to be vulnerable, because they use a process of subtraction, letting go of their own habitual patterns, so they can become a new character. Is this much different from what people want to do in therapy—become another version of themselves?

The old style of acting had students remember a real incident and bring it up to evoke a feeling. This can bring up real traumatic events from the past, and some of the events have not been processed, so the student often has a difficult time with the emotions. But newer styles of acting have the student do "what if" and imagine a scenario that would bring the emotion they want, and in the moment, they respond

II – ACTING

to it. This keeps it fresh, whereas the old way gets stale after a few tries, and it can be painful with an unprocessed emotion.

Might this be a softer way to process emotions if you are dealing with, let's say, a heartbreak?

1. Be in the real situation of the heartbreak, with the pain of what actually happened, and feel the mental, physical, and spiritual difficulty. (*I am so upset that person is gone. I can't sleep or focus on my life.* Etc.)
2. Rest.
3. Imagine a situation where "what if" somebody had a heartbreak. What would that person think, feel, and sense? How would they process it? (Maybe that person could have options, like talking to a friend, or going out in nature, or seeing a larger picture of life, and reasons for why things happen.)
4. Rest.
5. Go back to your own situation in 1. See if your outlook is any different.

EXPLORACISES

EX – How to Create a Character (or Yourself) from the Inside Out

Young actors think, "I need to look this way or that way to become this other person." But in truth creating a character isn't about how you *look*. It's more about:

1. What is happening inside you—how you see, hear, sense, and feel.
2. Inside, are you anxious or lighthearted? Your energetic state impacts how you see the world.
3. You can learn to shift your energetic state. Sometimes just by acknowledging it. Other times by processing inner feelings or sensations.
4. Another option is to think of someone you know.
5. What kind of energy do they have in their physicality? How they see and hear might be something that you never learned.
6. How does that energy affect how they relate in the world?
7. As you see how the energetic patterns in other people's physicality generate behavior, it enables you to alter the energy in your own body to create a character or to change your outlook. I can see, hear, sense, and feel another way. More possibilities and choices.

EX – Know Thyself

1. Larry Moss, the renowned acting coach, asks, "What would someone need to know about you to play you?"[1]
2. What am I proud of, ashamed of?
3. How do you speak? Softly, sarcastically, aggressively, shyly?
4. How did you become you?

II – ACTING

EX – Walking into a Room

1. Imagine walking into a room:
a. occupied by friends.
b. occupied by family.
c. occupied by a large group you are giving a presentation to.
2. What happens to the air as you walk in?
3. Next time you actually walk into a room of other people, notice what happens to the air around you. Do you take up more space? Or diminish the space?

> "A lesson I learned in drama school: the teacher asks, 'How do you be the queen?' And everybody says, 'Oh it's about posture and authority.' And the teacher said, 'No, it's about how the air in the room shifts when you walk in.'"
>
> —Meryl Streep

One of my clients played violin for the London Philharmonic. She told me what she remembered about Jessye Norman, the great opera singer. She said when Jessye walked out onto the stage and passed the instrumentalists, she felt the swish of Jessye's dress as she walked by, even though there was no actual contact.

EX – Acting and Effort

The moment of highest tension is the moment right before you begin anything. This is the moment you are likely to revert to old habits.

If you tend to fade (freeze), you will fade and then need to come alive.

If you tend to get hyper (fight or flee), you will get highly aroused and then need to calm down.

If you tend to collapse, you will need to be perky for it not to show.

1. As you tell any story, notice, *Am I overacting? Am I underacting?*
2. Notice the physical pattern: *Am I holding on? Am I letting go?*

When Heaven and Earth meet in synchronized embodiment, the amount of effort is just right.

III – MUSIC

Singing today includes physiological knowledge as well as psychological understanding. The question is not only *how does it sound?* but also *how does it feel?* This resonates with a quote from voice teacher Iris Warren: "I want to hear you, not your voice."

A singer or actor wants to convey the sound and movement of spoken word as an imaginative experience. They don't want to just utter or blare empty words. We receive auditory, olfactory, visual, tactile, or impressionistic images all the time from the nervous and fascial systems. The body is a global spring. The more sensory stimuli conveyed, the more holistic and clear the message. Then the purpose of performance is not just to entertain, but to heal. The performer feels the breath of life within that animates the emotions, and it spreads to the audience, the community, and beyond.

> "Breathing deeply the air common to all humanity, we may one day before it is too late—find and share words and stories that can save our universal souls."
>
> —*Kristin Linklater, master voice teacher*[2]

EXPLORACISES

EX – Let the Instrument Come to You

Most musicians pick up their instruments with excess tension, thus the phrase, "Grab your instrument." If not addressed, this grab carries into the playing.

Before picking up your instrument:

1. Become aware of the tendency to grab.
2. If possible, make another choice, one that does not include overly tensing your muscles, especially your hands, which want to remain suspended as part of the global tensional, tensegrity net.
3. This can create a type of vacuum in your hand that attracts your instrument.
4. Allow your instrument to come to you.
5. You can then be truly one with your instrument.
6. Play your music from here.

EX – Play Your Fake Violin (anyone can do this EX to feel a lighter arm)

1. Play your fake violin the way you would habitually play. Put it down.
2. Let your top hand rest on your bottom hand. Palm of the top hand on the back of the bottom hand.
3. Move your bottom hand up and down. As you let your bottom hand drop, your top hand drops also.
4. Let your bottom hand drop, and this time keep only your pinky of the top hand up as the bottom hand drops.

5. Do the same thing with the rest of your fingers, so that your bottom hand drops and the top fingers stay up. You are lightly holding your fingers up, and slightly pointing forward. Repeat with your other hand.
6. Explore moving all your fingers and both arms around with this slight pressure up and out on your fingers, and all the way up the underside of your arm.
7. See if your arm is not a little bit lighter.
8. Play your fake violin again.

EX – Play Your Instrument

Do these three steps, then play again.

1. Picture yourself as an hourglass, then check and see where your energy is. Is there more on top or bottom? If there is too much on top, imagine an hourglass and let the sand trickle down. If there is too much on the bottom, allow it to stream up.
2. Do a few Silent La La Las on your exhale (see Chapter 5). This extends your exhale by tricking the glottis into staying open, allowing your neck to release so your vagus nerve can enliven, bringing more ventral vagal activity to engage with yourself and your instrument.
3. Place your hands on your back ribs to feel your breath moving. This touches the kidneys and adrenal glands, which secrete adrenaline and cortisol. The warmth of your hands combined with the movement of the breath allows more ease for you to create and embody music.

Years ago, I was working with a jazz piano player. As he was improvising, I thought, *"That kind of sounds the same to me."* After we explored and found new pathways into his breathing and fascial matrix, he played again. It was completely different. I said to him, "Your improvisation is totally different now. What happened?"

He said, "After we gently and subtly shifted my habitual patterns, I heard new notes that I had never heard before, and I played them."

EX – In the Pocket

When musicians play exactly the right notes, they say the music is "in the pocket." It has a kind of universal, spontaneous connection—the essence of jazz.

1. What happens for you when you sing or play your instrument and everything is just right—the tone, the expression, the passion, and the intensity?
2. What happens in your physicality? Your emotions?
3. How is it when you do this with another or others?
4. How is it to be in the audience and listen, sense, and feel music played with this depth and dance of connection?
5. "In the pocket" implies that the music has a vibrational unity, unspoken but very palpable.

Uni-verse literally means one-song. We find the unity and the oneness in music, in relationships, and in life.

EX – Embodiment: Combining Brain Science and Functional Anatomy

Embodiment skills are the foundation from which musical skills grow. The skill to perceive and identify what you are doing, expressing the state of your body in the present moment, is invaluable for a performer. When you are embodied and healthy, you can create full and vital music. When you are not present in yourself and/or not well, there will be gaps and/or injury in your performance.

1. You want a clear picture of what you are doing in yourself, and how that relates to the world around you.
2. You want emotional ownership of what you are doing. Can you allow yourself to feel the depth of the material without falling to pieces in tears?
3. Are you willing to share what is happening in the depth of your soul to communicate the music with your audience?
4. These skills have brain systems that stand behind them.
5. You have *kinesthetic empathy* when music-making moves other bodies.

EXPLORACISES

THE HARMONIC SERIES

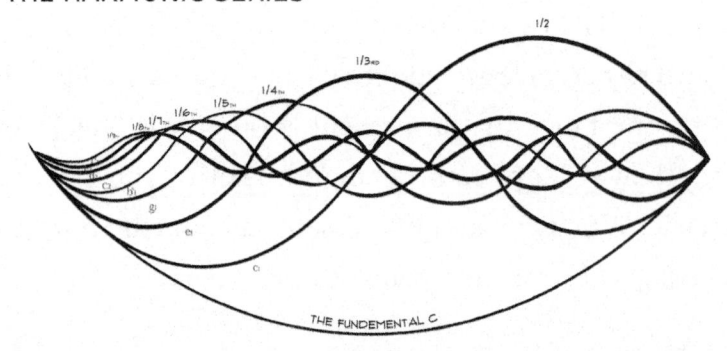

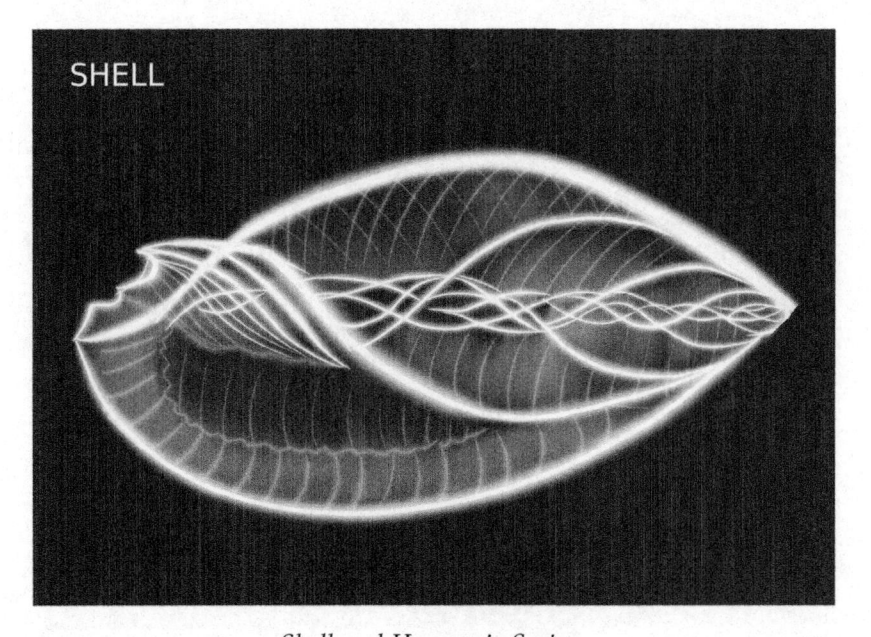

SHELL

Shell and Harmonic Series

III – MUSIC

Story of a Violin Player

A violinist got up and played in a master class. After she played, I asked why she played that piece. She said that she had played that piece for many years and now she was very anxious when she played it. She had played it for an audition about five years ago, and the audition did not go well, and since then she had felt anxious when playing that particular song.

That's understandable, but the interesting part occurred when I said to her, "I noticed when you played, you never looked up. You only looked at the strings." She had not noticed that. I asked her if she would be willing to play and explore looking up, even a tiny bit.

She began to play, and as she looked up, she jumped as if startled. I asked her afterward what happened. She said she was playing the piece, and then when she looked up, she saw the unpleasant faces of the panel from five years ago. She felt herself in that same uncomfortable audition room. Part of her was still living in that room and was not present to this room.

She had not realized that her vision of that audition room was still there and making her anxious. It was in realizing that the vision was still there that the change was able to happen. We did not deal directly with her anxiety. But we dealt with the root cause of the anxiety. It was a very interesting moment.

EXPLORACISES

EX – Sounds of Past Pain

Alfred Wolfsohn was a stretcher bearer in World War I. One can only imagine the sounds he heard while carrying injured soldiers to get help. After the war, Alfred had PTSD. He saved himself by making the sounds of pain that "he could not unhear." He let his body do the sounds of pain that lived inside him. This brought him out of dissociation and back into his body.[3]

1. Think of a difficult situation from your past.
2. Remember the sounds you wanted to make but could not. Remember what your body felt like.
3. Let your whole self express these sounds, either fully out loud if possible, or more completely with expressive breath and body movement.

EX – Singer's Mask

1. Singers today are often taught to put their sound in a mask in front of their face. This "places" the sound and creates a similar sound in all singers. Sound in front of the nose can sound limiting.
2. Do not place the sound. Don't put sound in a mask. The head, a resonating chamber, is three-dimensional with lots of space and holes for sound to vibrate in. This vibration ripples through the whole body, and the sound gets connected to the whole person. Your whole body sings.

EX – Voice and Pelvic Floor

The larynx and the pelvic floor evolved from the mesoderm, the middle of the three layers that differentiate during the early development of the embryo. The tissue rose up along both sides of the body for the two halves to meet in your throat.

1. Explore vibrating your larynx and feeling it down to your pelvic floor.
2. Move your lower torso and see if you feel your larynx move.

As you understand the fascial and tensegrity systems, of course, your whole system influences your voice.

EX – Vocal Presence includes:

1. Tone of voice
2. Physicality
3. Body language
4. Facial expression
5. Imagination
6. Spirit
7. Emotion
8. Bring them all to the stage!

EX – Singing and Effort

Recent research at the Lichtenberger Institute in Germany shows that vocal emission is an action caused 90 percent by involuntary muscles. This links it to the unconscious and therefore is little affected by voluntary action. This is opposite to what is taught in most vocal conservatories, where power, strength, and voluntary pushing are considered to be assets. According to the Lichtenberger training, maximum power can be released only in a low-pressure phonatory system, as the vocal cords develop their best potential for sound when it is emitted in largely effortless conditions.[4] Explore 1 and 2.

1. Sing with power and strength, while squeezing muscles for support. Stop and let it go.
2. Recognize your connection to the ground. Receive the support from the Earth, and allow your breath to flow, as you open your being to sing the effortless sounds that flow through you.

Of course, 2 is more aligned with Heaven and Earth in synchronized embodiment. It invites the divine vibration and frequency to bathe the cells and tissues of the singer and all who listen.

IV – TAKING THE STAGE

EX – For any performance:

1. Start with support. You always want to be connected to the planet and the air above. Without it, you are lost, untethered, separate, and alone.
2. As you are recognizing support, your environment is recognizing you. There is no separation. You vibrate together. Many singers "listen" to the hall before they start singing.
3. Create a field. A field of moving particles that shifts all the time. You want to be part of that, and to share that with your audience.
4. You have the ground, yourself, and the space around you. Now, step onto the stage!

EX – "Performance Anxiety"

1. In the Polyvagal Theory, any evaluation is seen as a threat of possible danger. There is certainly evaluation in performance. If you see the audience as dangerous, then you might run (legs shaking), fight (shoulders tighten), or try to appease them (lean forward), as you are in a sympathetic response pattern. Ideally for performance, you want to be in a ventral state, connecting through eyes, vocal prosody, and facial expression.
2. I have worked with students and clients with fears of performance for many years. It is well-known that fear of public speaking, by many polls, is bigger than the fear of death. The traditional historic reasons center on being excluded from the tribe. If one did something that shamed them in front of their tribe, they would be put out, exiled, and that might lead to death. Do we still have that mechanism in place? Or is it something else?

I recently was scheduled to speak at a large in-person conference. I prepare well for these, yet I still get a little excited/anxious in one form or another. Whatever form it takes, the symptoms usually disappear once I begin my presentation. Many performers tell me that they have a similar experience.

For this particular conference, there was a very large audience, about 2,000. Before my talk, my stomach was twisting and nauseous. As I started my presentation, I took time to connect with the audience, and something unusual began to happen. The tightening in my belly began to unravel, and in a way to send feelers of energy out that connected with the audience. It was like the early tightening was a preparation for this connection. It was a beautiful feeling that allowed a real flow between me and the audience. I think it allowed me to teach them what they needed, and they appreciated that with a standing ovation. Perhaps a new way to see performance anxiety is as a preparation or "wind-up" for performance connection.

    Try it.

CHAPTER 12

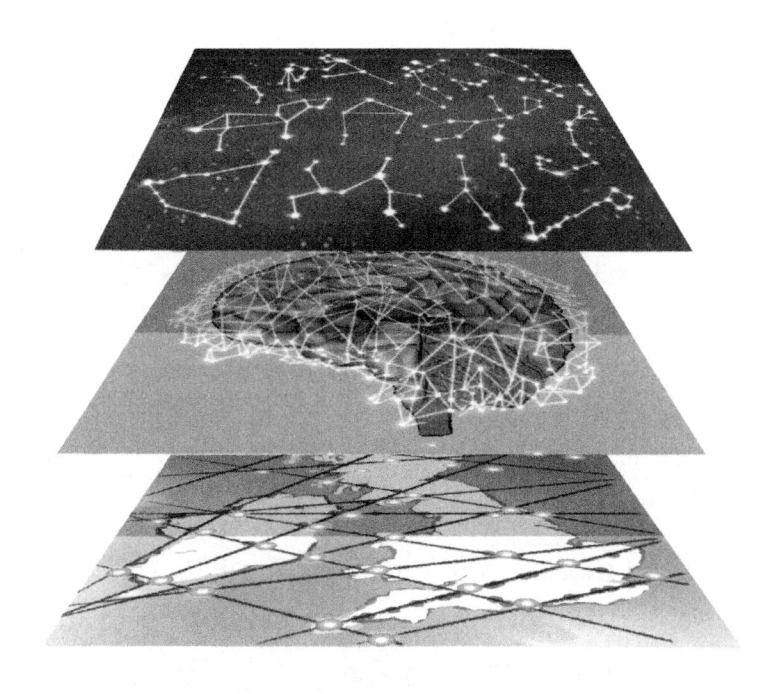

WE IS THE NEW ME

WE IS THE NEW ME

My interest in wellbeing and human potential continues to grow, beyond individual health to encompass the interconnectedness of all life. And I don't think we have any idea what that might include, as our awareness expands to recognize, as Rupert Sheldrake says, "Consciousness exists in everything."[1] Anybody reading this lives and shares the same Earth below our feet and the same Heavens above. We share the ground that we walk on, and the air that we breathe. Both include an element of movement: our feet connecting to and bouncing off the Earth, and our lungs taking in the swirling element of the atmosphere.

Breath and movement affect not only the body they are happening in, but also the air and Earth around them. My observations led me to this logical conclusion: If I am breathing and moving, it does not stop at me—it must spread to the Earth and Heavens. Or probably in reality it is the other way around. The Earth and Heavens move, and it spreads to me. Life is endlessly moving with some kind of order. If I have meridians, fascial pathways, breath and fluid running through me, so must the Earth and Heavens. And mine must meet with theirs. Thus is born the idea of Heaven and Earth meeting in synchronized embodiment. Where do they meet and how? What is the designated order?

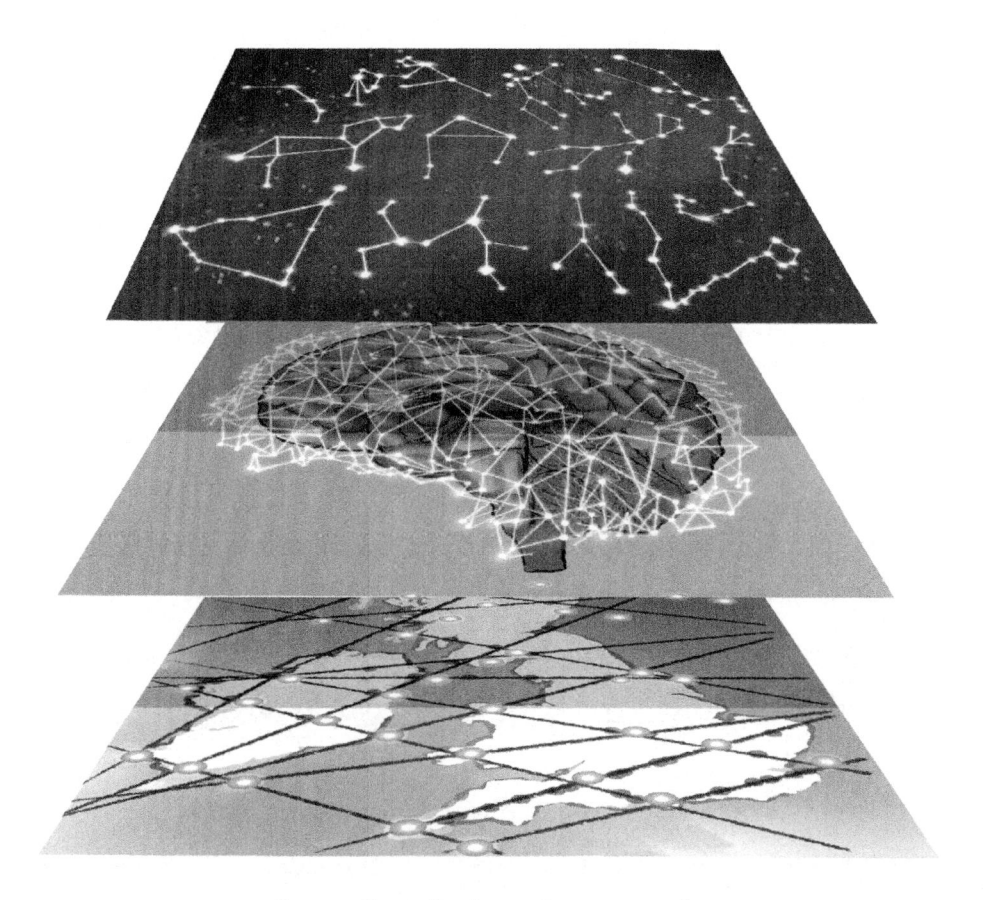

Energy lines, fascia, and cosmos stack

EX – Hierarchy and Heterarchy

1. A system that is hierarchical is ruled by an individual (or several) at the top. Historically, a wise, sacred leader was in control of a society or region. This leader had the wellbeing of everybody in mind for unity consciousness. As the epochs changed, in many cultures the leaders became corrupt, and life was more about separation and individual consciousness. Leaders were in power for their own benefit. In many realms of society, the hierarchical system became overbearing and unfair to anyone on the lower levels. Where do you see hierarchical systems in your life?

2. A system that is heterarchical has no top ruler or elite group. Control is distributed and shared, so some people have control now, and that can change so other people can make decisions at another time. The responsibility is shared, for better or worse. This is the atmosphere for group consciousness. Think of an orchestra with one conductor in charge versus a jazz jam session with no one in charge all the time, but the lead is shared at different times. Where do you see heterarchical systems in your life?

3. There is a well-known educational quote by Alison King—"from sage on the stage to guide on the side."[2] She is saying not to hammer information into our children, but to gently guide them to discover and learn. I might add to it: from sage on the stage to guide inside.

I once worked with an instrumentalist in a major US orchestra who shared the story that for one rehearsal the conductor was ill, so the practice went on without the conductor. My client told me that the orchestra played the piece better than they had ever played it, because they listened more to each other. All the members of the orchestra noted this. Of course, we don't know that such a connection would happen all the time. Sometimes jazz jams are great, and the lead flows seamlessly from one to another. Other times, the communication is off, and the jam is not so great. When would this idea work? When would it not work? More on how we are connected follows...

EX – Interstitium

1. Dr. Neil Theise, professor of pathology at the NYU Grossman School of Medicine, specializes in studying liver tissue to learn about disease. The tissue has many elements to it, including collagen, one of the components of fascia. He always saw the collagen as a wall with small cracks in the tissue but thought nothing of it. The medical community assumed that they were just cracks from dried-out tissue. In 2015, Dr. Theise observed live tissue with a new, very powerful scope and saw that the cracks were fluid-filled tubes and channels.[3] This was a huge surprise to him and his colleagues—and a major breakthrough in medicine, as before this, so many of the body's parts were thought to be independent and separate from each other, and not connected. Some parts valuable, others not. Imagine the fluid-filled tubes running through your whole body.
2. Before this, the medical community thought collagen was a useless, dense wall, and they threw it away in the garbage. The

new scope snaked through the body to see live tissue. The wall turned out to be more like a sponge—a three-dimensional honeycombed wall with fluid running through it. So alive! It surrounds every organ, nerve, blood vessel, bone, and muscle as it runs through the whole body. Picture this in yourself. The newly discovered system, itself an organ, was named *interstitium*.

3. Interstitium is part of the fascial system that we have been referring to, the body-wide communicator for the exchange of information. To make a clear distinction:

   The interstitium is the fluid-filled zone of fascial tissues. It creates a transition zone between the fatty layer (superficial) and deep fascia (tougher fascia surrounding muscles). We often conceptually bundle the interstitium and fascia together as connective tissue. All fascia is connective tissue, but not all connective tissue is fascia.

EX – The Oneness of It All

1. In the history of medicine, English scientist Robert Hooke in 1665 was one of the first to look through a microscope. He said human tissue looked like empty boxes and called them "cells" because they reminded him of the small rooms where monks lived in monasteries. A beautiful image. Who knew the word "cell" had a spiritual foundation? The cell, a basic unit of life, combined with other cells to form molecules, tissue, organs, and more. Nobody paid attention to the alive fluid that ran between, which allowed systems to communicate for a unified, healthy system. Modern life divides everything into parts and hierarchical jobs, creating a society and worldview of separation. But we are discovering

more heterarchical tendencies in the human system. Arthur Brock, social scientist, said, "We're in a paradigm shift. We're moving away from the scientific way of looking at the world as objects, to seeing a system-based world that's all about fluid, currents, connections, and relationships."[4] How do you see your life adjusting to this new conceptualization?

2. We are developing new rules in neuroscience and biomechanics, as well as new paradigms in physical, mental, and emotional health. We are seeing the unified, connected-system principle emerge more and more. Ecologists say the trees in forests are connected to one another with underground roots, trading information and nutrients across long distances. Mushroom networks intertwine their spreading, underground, horizontal mycelium. Nature is our teacher.

For us humans, connection is a biological imperative. Connection to ourselves and to each other. It is not just our cell phones that have connection, to our cars and computers… but we have a biological longing to connect to each other, even to those in different cultures. Western medicine is finding value in books about Traditional Chinese Medicine that are 5,000 years old. Wisdom from Indigenous cultures is reclaiming its rightful place in our world, as it is more widely recognized as valuable, instead of being wiped out. These healing traditions meet in roots underground. Community health organizations are popping up all over to help people find relational meaning and connection. We are now more than ever interested in helping to heal collective trauma and nourish the world with a habitat of love and compassion. Without it, we do not survive. Can you choose love and connection over fear?

3. In the Bible, Jacob said, "The Lord was always there, but I didn't know it." What else do we see now that was always there, but we didn't know it or see it? Now we see the interstitium that was always there before. In astronomy, we see the outer, dwarf planets that we never saw before. We are also recognizing the amazing powers of water that have always been there. The symbol of Aquarius is the water-bearer. Water sustains life for all of us. Water is full of consciousness. Water carries the light, which carries the information. Veda Austin, water researcher, takes a sunflower seed, puts it in water, chills it to crystal, and then sees a whole sunflower, not just the seed.[5] Water is able to read your optimal potential. Water is called God consciousness. What else about unity do we not see?

Maybe the balance of the divine masculine and the divine feminine needs to be restored to a seamless living whole. Maybe we can begin to see how connected we are as the human race—more we, less me. Too many years of patriarchy have left us with an unstable ecosphere, and an unsustainable lifestyle. Can we shift from being overly obsessed with material goods and our individual selves, and develop more respect and appreciation for the collective, and for spirit, prayer, and the mystery of the unseen? Perhaps then we will discover more about unity. The Age of Aquarius, is here with Heaven and Earth in synchronized embodiment.

> "Another world is not only possible—she's on her way. On a quiet day, I can hear her breathing."
>
> —*Arundhati Roy*

EX – Earth, Me, Heaven

1. Earth: A few years ago, I began studying dowsing with Rory Duff, geobiologist. Rory has mapped the low-frequency ley lines from the Earth's core. Where multiple energy lines meet is called a node. Visiting some of the nodes has been a profound experience. The energy provides a powerful combination of sacredness and earthly nature. At the sites, something is so present that you cannot see, but you can certainly feel. Note that we can see only 4 percent of reality. The rest of the electromagnetic spectrum is not observable to the human eye. At the node, while I was meditating, I was advised to put three pine needles on an old injury. I did. And I was urged to continue. But I had reservations about taking anything from the site because it was sacred. Nonetheless, I was told to take the three and then another cluster of three. And that was it. I thought that a little odd. I should probably have seven, not six. But six was the gift. As I was leaving later, I put everything down so I could put my hands together to pray in thanks. As I was praying and giving gratitude, a single pine needle fell on my little pile of six. I was given the seventh. I call it the miracle of the seventh pine needle. When I left the node, I thought, "It is the space between everything that I am aware of now." How would you feel that space?
2. Me: This brings us back to the expansive model that I have been studying, researching, teaching, observing, and writing about for many years (for example, in my previous book HUMANUAL): the space inside, outside, and in between—the expanded self. I had a dream a while back where I saw a field of white lace on top

of green grass. It was a beautiful image. When the wind blew, the sheet of white lace undulated in the breeze. Later that week, I was walking down the street, and I saw a green lawn with tiny white flowers. The white on green was the replica of my dream. The image continued. I felt in my physicality a quieting on the surface, but inside there was a lot of activity. Not anxiety-provoking, but very pleasant and spacious. I wondered if I was feeling the interstitium move. Then at night I closed my eyes to meditate, and there it was again—white-laced patterns over a dark background in the Heavens. Do your dreams show up in your daily life? The dream sparked me to write to Neil Theise, and ask, "Can you feel your own interstitium move?" To my surprise he wrote back, "Possible, I'm sure. But how to know? Tibetan pulse doctors tell me that is what the pulses are. So could fine attention to your own... maybe."

3. Heaven: I have always been fascinated with cosmology and the planets above us. I gave an oral report on "Why astrology works" when I was nine years old. Nobody, not my parents or my teacher, understood why I chose this topic. Like the Earth, the cosmos forms three-dimensional lines or pathways. Recent research on the ancient pyramids of Egypt implies that the pyramids were not just burial chambers, but portals between Heaven and Earth for humans to raise their consciousness. When I visited the Great Pyramid of Giza in 1978, I entered the king's chamber. I had had an awful stomach bug, but when I left the pyramid, my stomach was fine. The movement of the planets and stars are a major influence on human and galactic life.

WE IS THE NEW ME

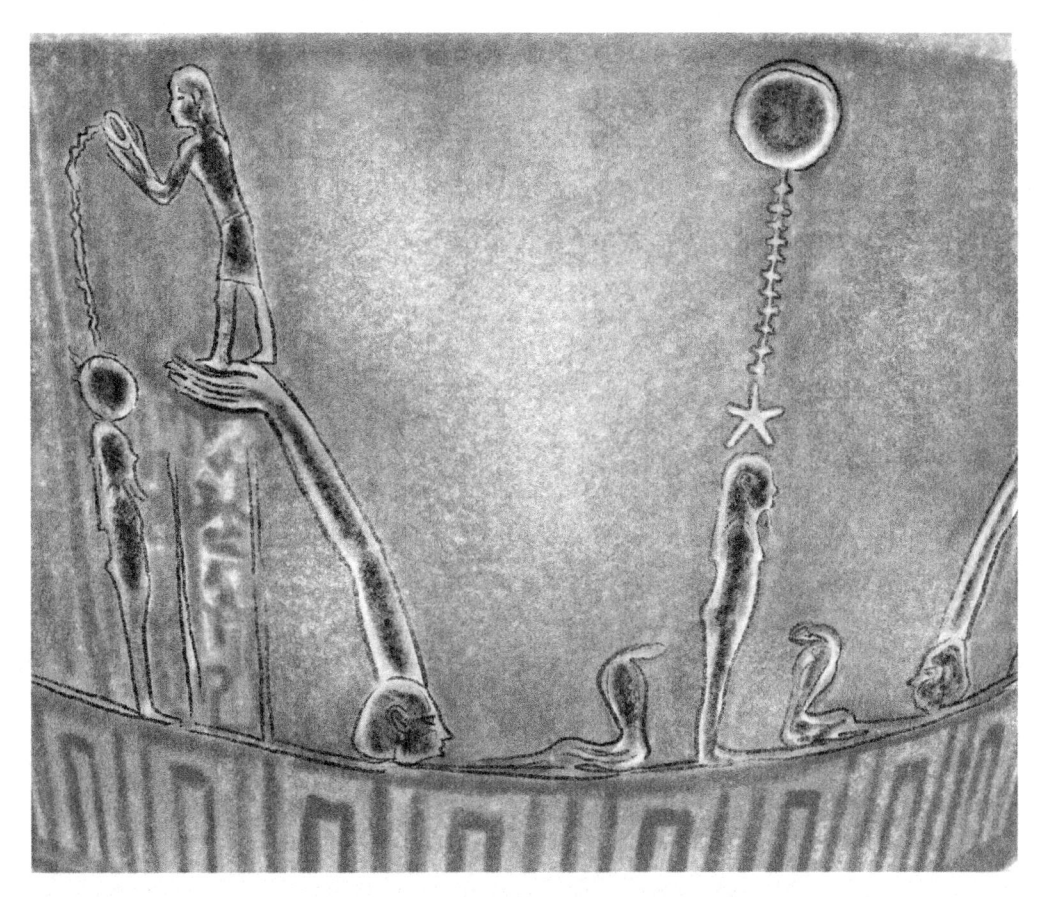

*Egyptian wall drawing, supported by Earth,
blessed by Heaven*

"As above, so below." We can be aware of the Earth's energy lines, our fascial network matrix, and the heavenly rotating bodies, all connected and parallel, Heaven and Earth in synchronized embodiment. The following EXploracises continue to lead us in this direction.

EXPLORACISES

EX – First Ponder

- There is a biological imperative to connect. These are the wise words of Dr. Stephen Porges. We do not survive on our own.
- From 4300 BCE to 2150 BCE, the astrological age of Taurus, in Mesopotamia, there were no weapons, fortified walls, or war that we know of today.[6]
- We are not here to undo what happened in the past. We are here to become conscious enough not to repeat it. Learn from what happened. If I am in a defensive state, I will put others around me in a defensive state. My task is to be in ventral vagal mode (at ease, and able to socialize) so that others are invited into that.
- You've got multi-layered imprints.
- Figure out how to live and share the land or share the graveyard beneath it.
- Walk beside someone instead of falling into their problems.
- Pine needles fall and turn brown. No weeds can grow there.
- You need to go against everything you are programmed to do.
- Offer curiosity, compassion, and presence instead of advising, controlling, or fixing.
- The opposite of shame? Maybe pride or acceptance.
- "When one tugs at a single thing in nature, one finds it attached to the rest of the world." —*John Muir*
- "We are walking each other home." —*Ram Dass*
- "Sovereignty of self and sanctity of relationship." —*Heather Ensworth, PhD*[7]

EX – Let's Rock

How did we as humans come to be? The story of the rib, the clay, and the mud never really resonated with me. Nor do I think that we all came from other planets, directly and fully formed to what we now call human. Maybe some of us did. But what I heard now is that we formed at the edge of the ocean and land, the ocean waters coming to the shore and then going back out, each time perhaps leaving some salt on the land, and that electrically charged salt became humans. What I like about it and what makes sense to me is the flowing in and out or back and forth. So many people rock back and forth all the time. It seems to be built in. Yes, it is comforting and soothing, as in rocking a baby, but it can also just be who we are and how we are made. We are not lumps of clay. We are moving, flowing, dynamic creatures. We rock and roll. Put on some up-tempo Elvis and try to stand still.

1. Rocking is a pattern that is one of our earliest vestibular experiences of movement. Notice when you rock.
2. Does your body remember the rhythm, motion, and speed of your mother/caregiver rocking you? Or were you put in one of those electric rockers for sleep or soothing?
3. Do you sometimes feel the rocking of anxiety and you can't sit still?
4. Do you rock to calm yourself?
5. Do you do inner rocking, like pulsing?
6. Or outer rocking, like swinging?

EX – Hidden Gems

We arrive as individuals, with multiple aspects of ourselves. Like a gem or cut stone, we have many facets, many different sides. Some facets shine in the light with brilliance, and others remain in the shadows. Your shadow is anything you don't love about yourself. Joy, love, shame, anger, and all their fellow characteristics take their turns jumping onto center stage. Most of us like to show our brilliance and not display our shadow, which was born from our adaptive patterns.

1. Name to yourself what you would least want someone to know about you. (I had to lie and exaggerate so people might listen. Or I had to hide to not be seen and hurt. Or I needed to be a predator for revenge.)
2. What happens in your physicality as you bring up these truths?
3. Check your head, heart, and belly.
4. Place your hand where needed, to bring compassion.
5. Remember the gem that you are as you allow all of you to arrive.

EX – Light and Light

Light as in light/dark and light as in light/heavy. Is there a correlation? Life begins with a zinc spark. There is a flash of light at the moment of conception. Upon fertilization, calcium increases, and zinc is rapidly released. When this happens, the zinc joins itself to small, light-emitting molecule probes. In other words, it creates a microscopic flash of light. We begin life with this flash of light.[8]

1. How much of that light do we maintain?
2. How do we stop that light?
3. At that first moment of conception, was there a perfect balance of light/heavy? When you make yourself heavy—not necessarily with weight, but maybe with thoughts, emotions, or attitudes—does that stop your flow of light?
4. You read in Chapter 6 that the heart is made of two spirals spinning in different directions. This includes a vortex in the left ventricle that is said to emit light rings. With training, these light beams can be transferred to another.[9]

> "When a guru or great teacher gives a Darshan, a golden flame leaves his/her heart center and opens yours."
>
> —*Rory Duff*

EX – We Walk in Shoes Too Small

1. Your soul has purpose and identity. Are you living it?
2. You have resources inside that you can find and utilize in life. Not always easy.
3. What supports you when all the supports you normally count on don't work?
4. What is your relationship to your own truth, your personal authority?
5. Fear and lethargy rob your life force. Only boldness releases you.
6. We serve life, not fear.

7. As you heal, the difficult triggers do less damage, and you recognize them sooner. And you outgrow their influence.
8. What wants to find expression through you? What is life bringing you now?

EX – Power and Essence

We are all born with essence: innate love, worthiness, courage, will, and more. When these get reflected back to us as children, we embody the power to move through life with confidence and rebound from difficulty when necessary. When they are not recognized and reflected back to us, the opposite is true.

1. How do you experience your own power?
2. Where and when do you lose power?
3. How do you experience your essence?
4. How has it carried you through the past?
5. What would your power look like if you had what you want?
6. What would you look like if you honored your own power?
7. What would life look like if your essential qualities were seen?
8. What if you saw everything that happened as if you had asked it to be that way?
9. Do you believe that you create your own reality?

Dr. Hans Selye, who coined the word "stress" in its modern usage, said,

> "The biggest stress of all is trying to be who you are not."

EX – Altered States Are at the Altar

1. Do you recognize the magic of daily life? The miracles? The synchronicities?
2. Catch and change the energy before it hits the physical dimension. We create from the invisible.
3. Keep the light alive. We are light beings. "Homoluminous."
4. You are fully human and fully divine.
5. Every thought, move, or sound that you make shifts the air around you, to move the planet, the stars, and other people. "The butterfly effect" refers to the potential effects and power of something as simple as a butterfly flapping its wings, which can cause a typhoon in another part of the world. *We* is the new *me*.
6. Start with self-acceptance versus self-improvement.
7. Can you have mind without judgment? We might call that serenity.
8. Do you choose fear or love?
9. Acceptance equals love.
10. What is it like to be you, if you are not judging yourself?
11. Embrace the vulnerability as you move life to the next stage.
12. Bow to your altar, whatever that may be.

EX – Animal / Human / Divine

1. Would your animal self ever think of going out on your own, and not considering the other members of the pack?
2. Would your human self ever think of gaining profit for only yourself, and not for the other members of the community?
3. Would your divine self ever think of liberating only yourself, and not the other members of humanity?

EX – As Above, So Below

I heard Professor Robert Temple, author of *A New Science of Heaven*, being interviewed by Heather Ensworth, PhD, astrologer and trauma therapist. He was talking about plasma and clouds between the Earth and the moon, a two-cloud system with the Earth and moon thrown in. Then he said something that really caught my attention. He said as you look at the moon, 60 degrees to the left and right are Lagrange points.[10] This is where the gravitational pull between the Earth and the moon equals zero. They balance each other out. The moon can't pull you toward it, and the Earth can't pull you toward it. The points are called L4 and L5. This is what knocked my socks off. Because anyone in the healing profession knows that L4 and L5 are Lumbar 4 and 5, the most common place for lower back pain and "slipped disk." It is an energetic roadblock that plagues many people. The talk had me wonder if this was some kind of balance point in humans. When you do the support EXploracises in Chapter 3 (EX – Stand with Support), with freedom at Lumbar 4 and 5, you can feel the weightless effect. As above, so below.

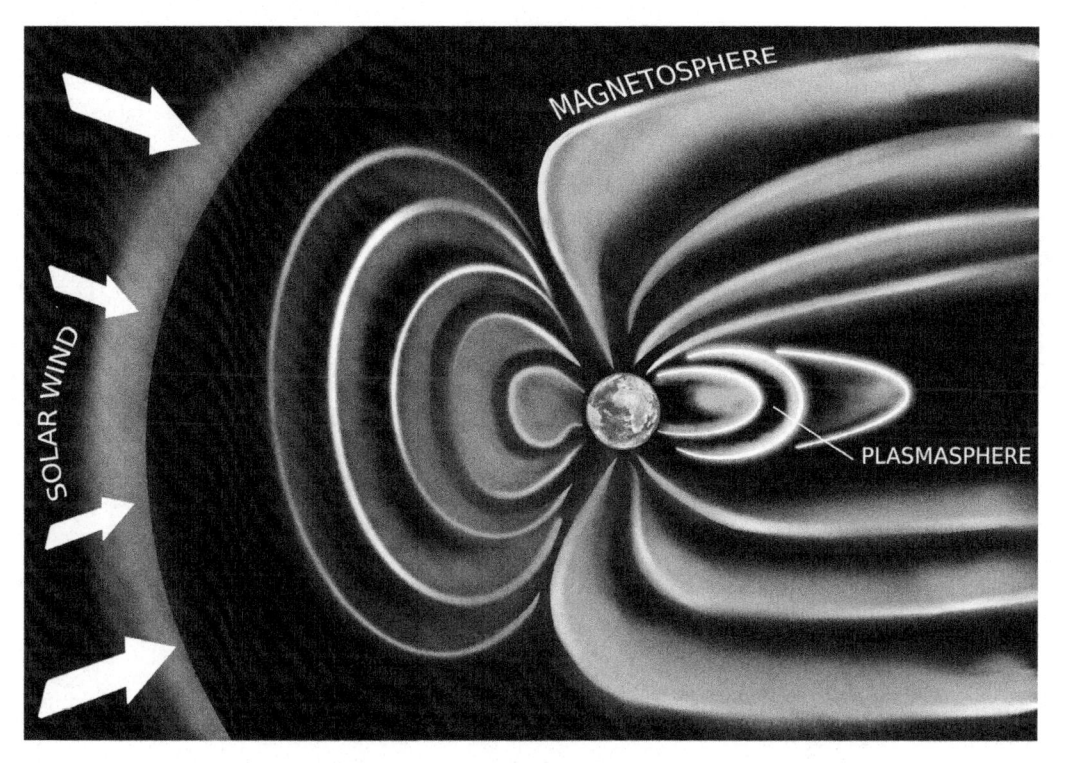

*Solar winds and Earth's magnetosphere
resemble our human form*

EX – Letting Go

Many self-help techniques suggest "letting go" in one form or another. But in truth, there is no need to let go of anything.

1. Can you let go of a thought?
2. Can you let go of a constriction?
3. Instead of trying to let it go, bring your attention to the constriction and see what happens. It releases a bit or seems to dissolve. You do not need to do the letting go. The you that would let it go is probably not the you that did the constriction in the first place. In other words, it was not conscious. You did not consciously put it in place, and you cannot consciously remove it by letting go.
4. Remember the wholeness of the fascial system.

EX – Snow Angel

1. Lie down and think of a snow angel. (This is when one lies on the ground in the snow and moves their arms up and down to create "wings" in the image when one stands up again.)
2. Imagine that you are now an Earth angel sinking into the Earth about a quarter inch.
3. You are leaving your mark. What might that look like?
4. What mark would you like to leave? Your archetypes might know the answer.

EX – Wise Words from Dr. Eva Eger, 96-year-old Holocaust survivor who became a therapist

1. "I understood perfectly in Auschwitz that I can neither escape nor resist, because if I climb to the guard, I will be shot, if I touch the barbed wire, I will die on the spot. And what is left to do? I was left to look for support in myself, because I did not have support outside of myself. The support within itself saved me."
2. "I told one of my patients: 'There were no antidepressants in Auschwitz.'"
3. "I often say that I have a wound, but I do not live in it: I worry about this wound, I do not ignore it, but I don't live in it and I do not focus my existence on it. I really hope I can push you to love yourself instead of victimizing yourself."
4. "I first realized we had a choice when I had to choose: to focus on what I lost or what I still have."[11]

EX – Choose Love

When I teach movement and breath from the expansive perspective, people's lives change, past holdings melt to the background, and a new sense of joy, purpose, and choice becomes available. Life seems to gel with the environment, instead of having to fight or fear it. Now when I see an image of the fascial system and the inner three-dimensional tubes and tunnels, I see the maps of the Earth's energy lines, and the maps of the planets and solar systems moving.

EXPLORACISES

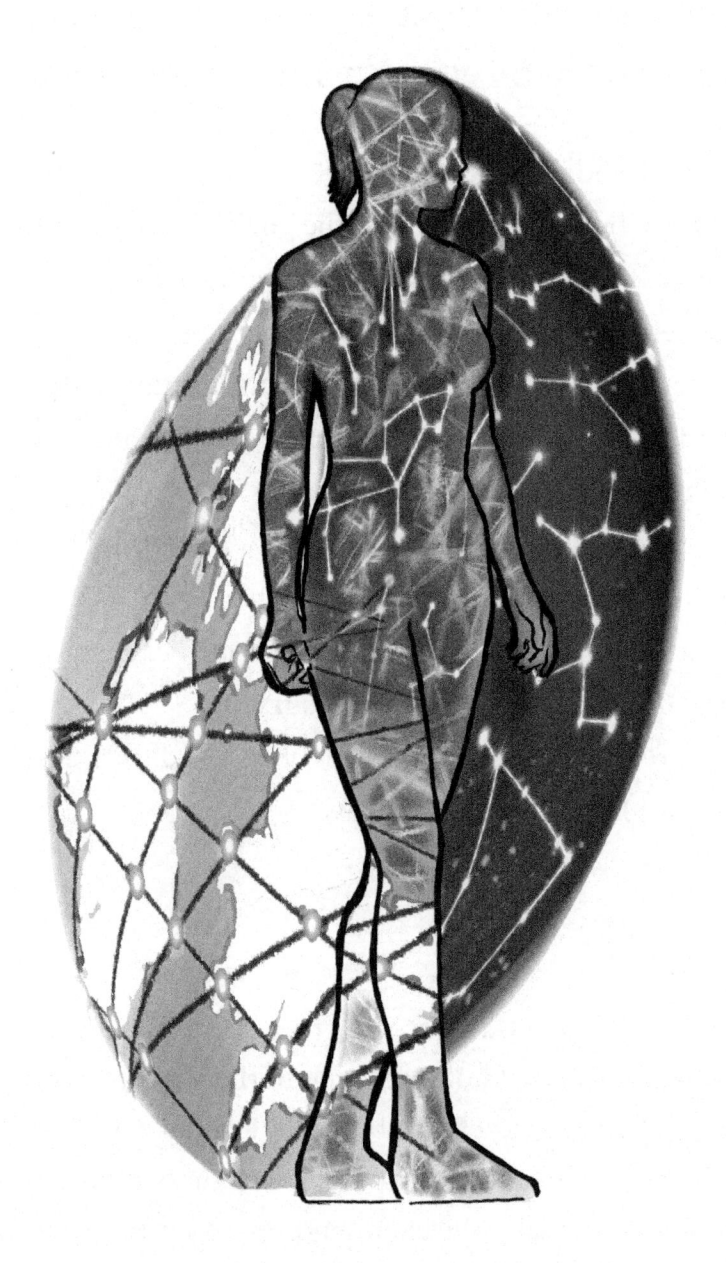

Energy lines, fascia, and cosmos together

Recognizing the unity of these systems restores wonder into our everyday experiences. We can understand the unity in ourselves and in our world, from the infinitesimal to the infinite. Our new world is emerging. Everything is consciousness. The Age of Aquarius is no longer just a song for hippies. It is a new paradigm for physicality, cognition, spirituality, medicine, our planet, and the universe, the interconnectedness of all things. Feel the wonder.

The implications are profound, providing insight into everything from the permeable boundaries of our bodies to the infinite nature of consciousness. Can we trade our limited, individualistic view for the expansive perspective of a universe that is dynamic, cohesive, and alive—a whole greater than the sum of its parts? Uni-verse as one-song. There is so much fluidity in our world and in ourselves. We live in a conscious cosmos. The exhilarating potential-expanding frontiers of human knowledge push us to choose love over fear and to coexist with a global grid of light. My wish is that we all have the strength, wisdom, and courage to go in this direction.

EXPLORACISES

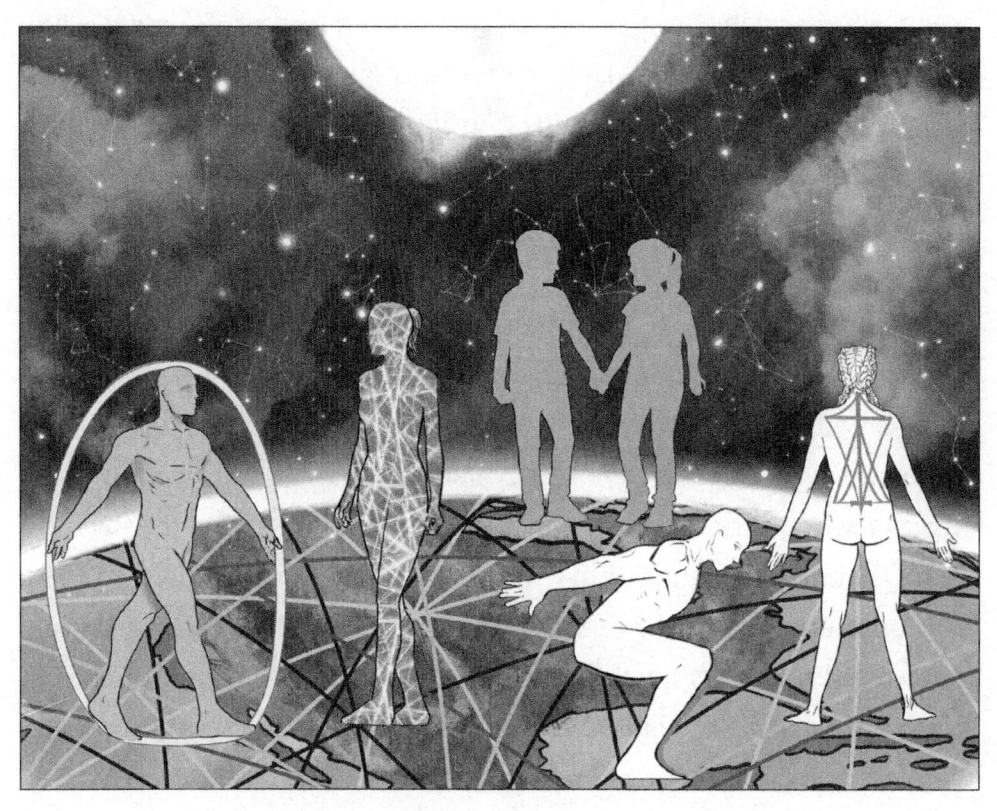

The big picture: energy lines, fascia, and cosmos together

ENDNOTES

All websites accessed in 2025.

Chapter 1: Wholeness, Tensegrity, and Fascia

1. Biotensegrity Archive. "Biotensegrity: a Model for the Heterarchical Integration of Biological Structure and Physiology." Uploaded November 24, 2024. YouTube video, 1:47:42. https://youtu.be/vBHi3YGvfIY?si=KQ2KhzMk-ycynRxf.
2. Levin, Stephen. "Biotensegrity & Dynamic Anatomy." Uploaded November 19, 2018. YouTube video, 34:36. https://youtu.be/jnpshtyvWr0?si=ivet0uP7Ew8PQm6O.
3. Kim, Ok-Hyeon, Tae Jin Jeon, Yong Kyoo Shin, and Hyun Jung Lee. "Role of Extrinsic Physical Cues in Cancer Progression." *BMB Reports* 56, no. 5 (April 20, 2023): 287–95. https://doi.org/10.5483/bmbrep.2023-0031.
4. "Move beyond Pain." Somatic Systems Institute | move feel live better easier. Accessed January 28, 2025. https://somatics.org/.

Chapter 2: Heaven and Earth Meet in Synchronized Embodiment

1. Rory Duff, Geologist, Geobiologist. Accessed January 28, 2025. https://roryduff.com/.
2. *"Gravity is the therapist,* levity the fool," *Structure, Function, Integration: Journal of the Dr. Ida Rolf Institute®*, Vol. 52, No. 1 (June 2024). https://www.rolf.org/docs/DIRI_Journal_June-2024_Interactive-Single_Pages_1.pdf.
3. Levin, Stephen. "Bouncing Bones." Uploaded March 15, 2024. YouTube Video, 10:30. https://www.youtube.com/watch?v=KtIwli80AqQ.
4. Pei-Jian Shi et al. "Capturing Spiral Radial Growth of Conifers Using the Superellipse to Model Tree-ring Geometric Shape." *Frontiers in Plant Science,* Vol. 6 (October 15, 2015), 856. https://www.ncbi.nlm.nih.gov/pmc/articles/PMC4606055/.
5. Special thanks to Muriel Barbery and Europa Editions for granting me permission to use this wonderful passage.

Chapter 3: Physicality

1. Tom Myers, speaking at the online Fascia & Chronic Pain Rescue Summit 2023, hosted by Shivan Sarna & Kelly Kennedy. Video not available.
2. Almaas, A. H. *Essence with the Elixir of Enlightenment: The Diamond Approach to Inner Realization*. Newburyport: Red Wheel Weiser, 1998.

3. Jones, Frank Pierce. *Body Awareness in Action: A Study of the Alexander Technique.* New York: Schocken Books, 1976. Reprinted as *Freedom to Change,* London: Mouritz, 1997.
4. Polatin, Betsy. *HUMANUAL, An Epic Journey to your Expanded Self.* Cardiff-by-the-Sea, CA: Waterside Productions, 2020.
5. Lanius, Ruth. Lecture, Trauma Research Foundation International Conference, Boston, MA, 2015.
6. Brown, Walter A. "Acknowledging Preindustrial Patterns of Sleep May Revolutionize Approach to Sleep Dysfunction," *Psychiatric Times,* May 26, 2006.
7. Calamassi, Diletta, and Gian Paolo Pomponi. "Music Tuned to 440 Hz versus 432 Hz and the Health Effects: A Double-Blind Cross-over Pilot Study." *EXPLORE* 15, no. 4 (July 2019): 283–90. https://doi.org/10.1016/j.explore.2019.04.001.
8. Porges, Stephen, and Anthony Gorry. "The Sound of Science." Sonocea. Accessed January 29, 2025. https://www.sonocea.com/.

Chapter 4: Taking EXploracises to the Next Level

1. Ensworth, Heather. Interview with Ron LaPlace. "Sacred Geometry, Sound Healing and Opening Our Illuminated Hearts." Uploaded August 17, 2024. YouTube video, 1:00:22. https://youtu.be/YNf9nuVQmnQ?si=3H0vgIw_Pjf0bR3b.
2. Cash, Johnny. "In Your Mind." Recorded 1995. Track 2 on *Dead Man Walking.*
3. Dart, Raymond. "The Attainment of Poise." *South African Medical Journal* 21 (February 8, 1947): 122.
4. https://neuroaffectivetouch.com/.

5. Hedley, Gil. "Nerve Stitches: Learn Integral Anatomy with Gil Hedley." Uploaded February, 26, 2023. YouTube video, 4:30. https://www.youtube.com/watch?v=CN62ZqQqdV4.

Chapter 5: Breath

1. Stough, Carl. *Breathing: The Source of Life.* New York: Stough Institute, 1996. DVD.

Chapter 6: Heart

1. Hedley, Gil. "Unwinding the Heart Center." Uploaded January 15, 2021. YouTube video, 4:30. https://www.youtube.com/watch?v=MbOyozg_GTs.
2. "HeartMath Institute." HeartMath Institute. Accessed January 29, 2025. https://www.heartmath.org/.
3. Darwin, Charles. "General Principles of Expression - Concluded." In *The Expression of the Emotions in Man and Animals*, 69, 1872.
4. Ensworth, Heather. Interview with Ron LaPlace. "Sacred Geometry, Sound Healing and Opening Our Illuminated Hearts." Uploaded August 17, 2024. YouTube video, 1:00:22. https://youtu.be/YNf9nuVQmnQ?si=3H0vgIw_Pjf0bR3b.

ENDNOTES

Chapter 7: Spirit and Meditation

1. "Alexander Technique and Spirituality," *Direction* magazine (2005).
2. *HUMANUAL* is my previously published book and a practice for accessing one's inherent function and true nature. It is a unique and comprehensive approach to self-knowledge and self-improvement. Polatin, Betsy. *HUMANUAL, An Epic Journey to your Expanded Self.* Cardiff-by-the-Sea, CA: Waterside Productions, 2020.

Chapter 8: Emotion

1. Wilhelm, Richard, trans. *The Secret of the Golden Flower: A Chinese Book of Life.* Victoria: Must Have Books, 2023.
2. Private conversation with Rory Duff about Goethe's fairy tale, "The Green Snake and the Beautiful Lily" (2023).
3. Porges, Stephen. Lecture. Cape Cod Summer Institute, 2018.
4. Maté, Gabor. Lecture. Wisdom of Trauma Retreat, online, 2021.
5. Carter, Sue. Lecture, Belfast Trauma Summit, Belfast, Ireland, June 2024.
6. Goelz, Donnalea. "Benefits of Somatic Intervention Informed by the Polyvagal Theory." Masters Trauma Conference, Oxford, England, 2024.
7. Cotler, Steve. "Little Songs on Big Subjects." Steve Cotler, February 9, 2022. https://stevecotler.com/2009/03/08/little-songs-on-big-subjects/.

Chapter 9: The Vagus Nerve and the Polyvagal Theory

1. Porges, Stephen W. *The Polyvagal Theory: Neurophysiological Foundations of Emotions, Attachment, Communication, and Self-regulation.* New York: W.W. Norton, 2011.
2. Porges, Stephen. Lecture. Belfast Trauma Summit, Belfast, Ireland, June 2024.
3. LaPierre, Aline. Private conversation, 2023.
4. Karsenty, Gerard. "Osteocalcin: A Multifaceted Bone-Derived Hormone." *Annual Review of Nutrition* 43, no. 1 (August 21, 2023): 55–71. https://doi.org/10.1146/annurev-nutr-061121-091348.
5. Polatin, Betsy. "The HUMANUAL Polyvagal Smile." In *Somatic-Oriented Therapies: Embodiment, Trauma, Polyvagal Perspectives.* W. W. Norton & Company, 2025.

Chapter 10: Trauma

No notes.

Chapter 11: Performance

1. Rodenburg, Patsy. Interview with Larry Moss. *Patsy Rodenburg – Craft, Sweat, and Joy.* Podcast audio, April 8, 2024. https://podcast.patsyrodenburg.co.uk/2309772/episodes/14827933.
2. Linklater, Hamish, and Andrea Haring. "In the Company of Kristin Linklater and Her Natural Voice." AMERICAN THEATRE, June 17, 2020. https://www.americantheatre.

ENDNOTES

org/2020/06/16/in-the-company-of-kristin-linklater-and-her-natural-voice/.

3. Anderson, Kaya. "The Transmission of Alfred Wolfsohn's Legacy to Roy Hart." Centre Artistique International Roy Hart, January 2, 2022. https://roy-hart-theatre.com/shop/the-transmission-of-alfred-wolfsohns-legacy-to-roy-hart/.
4. "Lichtenberger Institut Für Angewandte Stimmphysiologie." Accessed January 31, 2025. https://www.lichtenberger-institut.de/.

Chapter 12: We Is the New Me

1. Sheldrake, Rupert. "Angels and the Festival of Michaelmas." Uploaded September 23, 2024. YouTube video, 23:50. https://youtu.be/ooaY1NHPSWI?si=4BFY818UDFS5umX4.
2. King, Alison. "From Sage on the Stage to Guide on the Side." *College Teaching* 41, no. 1 (January 1993): 30–35. https://doi.org/10.1080/87567555.1993.9926781.
3. Theise, Neil. "The Interstitium." *Radiolab.* Podcast audio, November 17, 2023. https://radiolab.org/podcast/interstitium.
4. Brandel, Jennifer. "Invisible Landscapes." *Orion Magazine*, November 16, 2023. https://orionmagazine.org/article/interstitium-scientific-discovery-anatomy/.
5. "The Secret Intelligence of Water." vedaaustin.com. Accessed January 31, 2025. https://www.vedaaustin.com/.
6. "The Marija Gimbutas Collection." OPUS Archives and Research Center. Accessed January 31, 2025. https://www.opusarchives.org/marija-gimbutas-collection/.

7. "Heather Ensworth, Ph.D. - Rising Moon Healing Center." Rising Moon Healing Center, November 24, 2024. https://risingmoonhealingcenter.com/.
8. LaPierre, Aline. Lecture. NeuroAffective Touch training, 2024.
9. Duff, Rory. Newsletters, February 2022. https://roryduff.com/news/.
10. Ensworth, Heather. "Interview with Robert Temple About his Book, *A New Science of Heaven.*" Uploaded February 1, 2023. YouTube video, 1:04:48. https://www.youtube.com/watch?v=O4_l56FYfrk.
11. Source: https://ukrainky.com.ua.

ABOUT THE AUTHOR
Betsy Polatin

An internationally recognized breathing/movement and somatic trauma-resolution specialist, Betsy Polatin, MFA, SEP, AmSAT, was a professor of Theater and Music at Boston University's College of Fine Arts for 25 years. She is the author of the bestseller *HUMANUAL, an Epic Journey to your Expanded Self* (2020).

Her background encompasses 50 years of movement education and performance, as well as training in music, dance, yoga, meditation, trauma resolution, and the broader healing arts. Her teaching experience includes Berklee College of Music, Touch and Movement in Trauma Therapy, Muscular Therapy Institute, Kripalu, The Embodiment Conference, Tanglewood Music Festival, and the Opera Institute of Boston. Betsy has taught Master Classes for the Psychotherapy Networker, Performing Arts Medicine Association, Bessel van der Kolk's International Trauma Conference, Masters Events Oxford, Belfast Trauma Summit, International

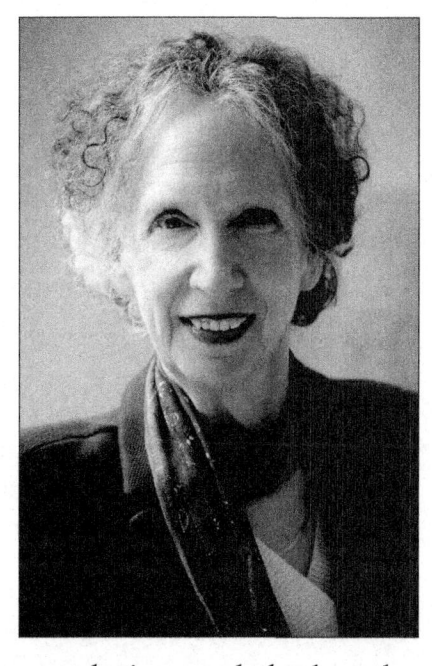

Yoga Conference in Japan, US Association for Body Psychotherapy, Pittsburgh Symphony Orchestra, Spiritual communities, Children's Hospital, Boston Ballet, Sports Medicine clinics, and the Science and Nonduality Conference—in the United States, Europe, Australia, India, Japan, and Korea.

Since 2016, she has been co-teaching traveling workshops, themed "Trauma and the Performing Artist" and "Trauma in the Public Eye," with Peter A. Levine, PhD. She also teaches "Returning to Ourselves, the Wisdom of Trauma," with Dr. Gabor Maté.

Betsy leads international trainings where she presents her unique and revolutionary fusion of ideas: scientific knowledge combined with ancient wisdom and intuitive human creativity. This work helps people recognize their habitual patterns, which are often charged with unconscious commitment. Once these patterns are brought to awareness, deep change can happen on many levels, as the life force resumes and strengthens. Her work is greatly influenced by the teachings of Spiritual and Meditation Masters.

Betsy's book *The Actor's Secret* (2013) was featured on ABC TV and Fox News, received rave reviews, and is now a recommended textbook in many performing arts schools. She is the author of a chapter in the Norton Professional Series book, *Somatic-Oriented Therapies: Embodiment, Trauma, Polyvagal Perspectives.* As a well-known educator, she has published numerous articles in the *Huffington Post*. Betsy has a training/nontraining course and maintains a private practice in Malibu Canyon, California and internationally online.

Please visit: betsypolatin.com

Printed in Great Britain
by Amazon